# Chasing the Light

*Julia Boggio*

# Chasing the Light

## A Novel

### Julia Boggio

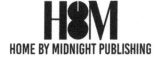

**H8M**

HOME BY MIDNIGHT PUBLISHING

To request permissions, contact the publisher at hbmpublishingUK@gmail.com.

Paperback: 978-1-7392151-3-2

First edition.

Cover design: Bailey McGinn

Library in Congress Cataloguing-in-Publication has been applied for.

*For Sarah Gillman*
*and all the other*
*warrior women out there*

1

———

FRANCESCA HATED WEDDINGS.

Number one: they were a waste of money. Even just being a guest these days was a major investment: the outfit, the hat, the hotel, the gift, not to mention the hen and stag dos. Attending two weddings per year would bankrupt most twenty-somethings. And the couples...so many started their married life in debt because they spent too much money on items like personalised wedding favours destined for landfill.

Number two: the drama, in the form of (but not excluded to) drunken brawls, Bridezillas, jealous bridesmaids, horny groomsmen, and over-bearing parents.

Number three: weddings were *boring*. Same thing every time. The couple says the vows before having a meal and making everyone sit through speeches downloaded from the Internet. Then they do a crappy dance and cut a dry cake that costs more than a holiday to Ibiza. And sometimes, there were fireworks.

Number four, and the thing Francesca hated most about weddings: she'd probably never have one herself.

She looked up at the wooden pub sign, creaking in a light summer breeze: The Bleeding Hart, featuring a charming picture of a deer with its insides ripped out by a smiling hunter. What a fitting place to meet the groom and his party, a group of virile men celebrating the thrill of conquest. She sympathised with the deer.

An uncomfortable ache radiated from her middle, and she inhaled deeply through her nose. She made a little O with her mouth and pretended to blow out a candle—a technique she'd learned from a YouTube video. Apparently it was a breathing technique that helped women in labour. It helped Francesca, too. Helped her breathe through the pain that rippled through her, even with the co-codamol taking the edge off.

Frowning at the sign, she readjusted the bag full of video equipment weighing down her shoulder.

Eight hours. Only eight hours and it would be done. Eight hours and she could go home to curl up with a hot water bottle.

As she worked up the resolve to go inside, a man in a football jersey stubbed out a smouldering cigarette on the pub wall and chirped at her, 'Cheer up, love. It might never happen.'

She stopped and cocked her head to the side. *Be nice, Francesca,* she told herself. *He's just trying to flirt with you in his own twisted, ineffectual way.*

'Fuck off, twat face,' she said.

*Close enough.*

Francesca lifted her lips into a practised smile and yanked the door open.

Friendly chatter washed over her as she entered the swanky East End pub. It was working hard for that historic public house look: dark wooden beams treated to seem three centuries old, paintings of men in wigs with their hunting dogs acquired from ye olde boot sale, lots of brass. *Tossers.* As a woman, the decor almost repelled her. Cast ye out, oh child of Eve! Here be the den of men.

Her eyes landed on the groom straightaway: dark hair and manic eyes, standing at the gleaming mahogany bar with some Dutch Courage in hand, surrounded by men in matching grey tails, pink cravats, and top hats. They looked like an advert for Moss

Bros. So original. She pursed her lips hard to stop her eyes from rolling.

She walked towards him. As she got closer, the stale beer smell oozing from the carpets was replaced by a soupy mix of colognes. 'Hey, Robert.'

'Francesca!' He kissed her on each cheek, which she tolerated. She wasn't a fan of other people invading her space.

'How are you feeling?' She smiled like she cared.

'Oh, you know. Having my last drink as a free man.' He laughed. She laughed.

'Great. Um, so I just need to mic you up.'

She loathed this part. It involved feeding a wire through the groom's jacket and attaching a lavalier under his corsage. She always performed the manoeuvre as professionally as possible, with minimal contact, and yet Francesca was willing to bet there would be at least one lewd comment from the groom's party.

With the mic in place, she asked the groom to do a routine soundcheck. 'Robert, could you tell me what you had for breakfast?'

She could practically feel it coming when the best man leaned in and said, 'Jenny!' He slapped the groom on the back, and Robert threw Francesca an embarrassed smile while snickering along with his mates.

*So clever, you see, because Jenny is the bride. Get it?* She bit her tongue. How many hours were left until she could go home?

Turning the groom towards the door, she flipped up the tails of his morning coat, so she could attach the mic pack to his waistband. The metal clip could be sticky, so she had to fiddle with it to get it open. As she did that, the tails of his coat kept slipping down to cover it, making her job harder.

Just as she managed to get it on, a new, deep voice joined the crowd. 'Hi, Robert. All good?'

'Krish!' said the groom. Francesca froze, her eyes fixating on the way the back of the groom's jacket rippled as he shook hands with the newcomer.

Her heart pumped adrenaline through her. She'd known this day would come. The wedding industry was small. It was inevitable that one day she'd find herself shooting a job alongside her ex-boyfriend.

She just wished it wasn't today.

For a few moments, she hid behind the groom. He was taller and wider than she was, giving good coverage for her petite frame. She did her breathing exercise again, this time to calm her nerves, and scraped back her straight, dark brown hair. The memory of the night she broke up with Krish five years ago forced itself to the forefront of her mind.

'I've met someone else,' she'd said. The lie she'd told him to cover up her other, bigger lie.

The look on his face had almost killed her, but it was the only thing she could think of that would be guaranteed to end the relationship, aside from moving to Timbuktu. They'd dated for six months, the point where a relationship either got serious or it didn't. Conversations about the future and buying property together and having kids...well, those had been on the increase. That's why she'd walked away.

In another lifetime and another set of circumstances, she could be his wife by now. The thought made her eyes sting. She blinked rapidly to hurry the tears away. No time for that. She had a job to do.

Francesca sucked in a steadying breath. She wondered if he'd still look the same. Fixing another false smile on her face, she stepped out from behind the groom.

'Hey, Krish.'

Time stopped as their eyes connected. Sexy black hair that ran through her fingers like silk, its scent masculine and sweet at the same time. Those dimples on his cheeks. Burnt umber in his gaze. In those seconds, she remembered kisses and caresses and laughter. Cinema nights and dinners and trips to the beach. The calluses on his hands and the warmth of his skin. How nibbling his earlobe drove him crazy. How his hair tickled the inside of her thigh as he licked—

4

Her cheeks flamed.

'Francesca.'

No greeting. No surprise. Just her name. As though ex-girlfriends turned up all the time. *Ooh, burn*, she thought.

'You two know each other?' asked the groom before taking a long sip of his beer.

'Old friends,' said Krish, breaking eye contact with her to turn away and twiddle with the settings on his camera.

Two could play at that game. He wanted to pretend that they were just 'old friends'? Fine. She would be the picture of polite professionalism. *Krish who?*

She reached into her kit bag and drew out the second mic for the best man. She repeated the exercise of attaching the lavalier to his lapel and asking him what he'd eaten for breakfast. She didn't even react when his eyes flicked up and down her body before answering, 'Hot, sticky buns.'

FRANCESCA STILL NEEDED TO MIC UP THE FATHER OF THE BRIDE, A good excuse to get away from Krish and the pre-wedding testosterone fug of the groomsmen. She asked Robert where to find his soon-to-be father-in-law.

He flinched, and a twinge of something like fear flitted across the groom's face and was gone. 'He's around the corner. Pinstripe suit. Hat. Dark glasses. Can't miss him.'

*Weird.* She packed up her bag, extricated herself from the boys, and walked around the perimeter of the bar. She used the distance to take a better look at Krish.

He had changed, and he hadn't. Obviously he was still tall: six foot three to her five foot two. She remembered how he used to lean down when he kissed her. His black hair was longer now, and sexier, with a slight wave. When she'd met him, his hair had been short, businesslike. He'd been thinking of moving from law, which he didn't love, to photography, which he did. It was she who encouraged him to make the jump. Her gaze moved to the place formerly occupied by his dimples, now hidden beneath a short, manicured beard. But his eyes were the thing that she missed most: so bright and full of humour, except of course when he looked at her today.

At least he didn't have the monopoly on change. She'd done her fair share, too. After she'd left him, she decided to improve her symptom management. She'd hired a nutritionist and a personal trainer, which helped her become better at regulating her weight. The acne was also under control, and when it wasn't, her improved make-up skills helped.

Lost in her own thoughts, she was surprised when a bald, thick-set man in a black suit suddenly blocked her path.

'What's your business?' he demanded.

She took a step back. Who was this man? 'Watch it, Rock. I'm here to mic up the bride's father.' When he stared blankly, she raised her eyebrows and said, 'I'm the videographer.'

'Stay here.' The man swaggered over to an older gentleman sitting at a table with two friends, also in their sixties. The gentleman wore a Fedora and a navy pin-stripe suit: the father. He had on those glasses that could transition from sunlight to indoors, the lenses hovering somewhere in between making it hard to see his eyes. The Rock mumbled something in the father's ear, then strutted back to her. 'You're alright,' he said.

'Gee, thanks.'

Francesca stepped up to the table and introduced herself.

'Larry,' the father said, extending a hand with an oversized golden signet ring facing up, like he expected her to kiss it. At the last moment he flipped his hand sideways to envelop hers, squeezing her knuckles together as he shook it. She kept her face impassive. She'd met this kind of man before: the kind who confused dick-swinging with just plain old being a dick.

The two other men introduced themselves with milder handshakes.

She just wanted to get this done. 'Can you stand up so I can mic you?'

'Alright, love. Plenty of me to go around,' he said in a strong Cockney accent. The other two men laughed, although she wasn't quite sure she got the joke. Larry unfolded to his full height, not much taller than her and twice as wide. His cologne unfurled around her, a pungent soapy smell ending on a hint of cloves. She hated it.

Trying not to gag, she unwound the wire and asked him to undo his jacket. She clipped on the lavalier, feeding the wire under his coat.

Her eyes flicked to Krish, who was photographing the groomsmen one by one near a big picture window. Just before they'd broken up, he secured an assistant position with Connor Knight—the world's best wedding photographer—and she'd been making documentaries. After they broke up, her finances pushed her to walk away from documentaries and give videoing weddings a try. She needed money fast. Aside from that, the schedule worked better with her body's specific needs.

God, Krish filled out a suit well. He looked even more muscular than when they'd dated. She wondered if he had a girlfriend—or worse—if he was married. The thought made her frown.

The father said something to her and she refocused on him. 'Sorry?'

'I don't like this mic, love. Too big. It'll ruin the line of my suit.'

She didn't need this bullshit right now. 'Don't worry. Your arse does that already.'

It took a moment for her to register the silence and realise, with a shock, she'd spoken out loud. Slowly, she looked up.

The two men sat deathly still, their eyes darting between her and the father of the bride. Taking her cue from them, she also froze, her fingers hovering on the mic pack at the back of Larry's trousers.

Fuck her and her big mouth. In normal circumstances, she was good at hiding her cheeky side. Krish's sudden appearance had put her off her game. She could feel the hulking presence of the Rock behind her.

An apology stuck like wet cotton balls in her throat.

Larry's head swivelled towards her at a glacial pace, the faint outline of unamused eyes visible through his tinted glasses. He regarded her for a second that felt as long as a Peter Jackson film.

And then he laughed.

'Ha! That's a good one. I like you. She's funny.'

The other men exchanged a relieved look and also laughed, the tension dissolving as quickly as it had come.

She really did not need this extra stress today. Every wedding was already a game of chance for her: would she wake up that morning free of pain, or would her broken body decide to unleash hell? She took on a maximum of three wedding bookings per month and spent the rest of her time in the editing room. Three days per month. Just three days where her body needed to not be an arsehole.

Today, she'd lost the game. All she could say was thank god for painkillers.

She moved away from the men and found an empty table where she could prep her video equipment.

'Everything okay?'

She jumped to find Krish standing behind her, his film-poster handsome face creased with concern. Turning back to her bag, she said, 'Yeah. Why?'

'I thought I saw some tension with the father...'

'It was nothing. Anyway, I can handle myself. Thanks.' Krish had always had an overdeveloped Lancelot Complex. He liked to be the knight in shining armour, but she was beyond saving. She wished he would go away and let her get on with her work.

He didn't. Lowering his voice he said, 'Do you know who the bride's father is?'

Taking out her monopod, she extended the leg with a snap and secured it. 'Larry? I don't know. A retired construction worker? He has the build for it.'

Krish huffed a laugh. 'He does love a shovel, but not for construction.' As he leaned towards her, she could smell the lemony soap he'd used that morning. When they'd been together, they used to love a good shower. Running the soap over each other's bodies, the frictionless way she would glide up his torso when he lifted her to his height, her legs wrapped around his middle, her back pressed against the cool tiles.

She ignored the flutter in her stomach.

'Larry, as you call him, is also known as Larry "Chuckles" Bonneface. He used to dispose of bodies for the McGinny crime family.'

What a mood killer. Her eyes went wide and she couldn't help glancing towards the sexagenarian and his cronies. 'No bloody way.'

'Don't look at them!' Krish said in a hushed tone, putting his hand on her arm and turning her away. Her skin blazed under his touch. She shook him off more aggressively then she meant to. A flicker of hurt passed over his eyes before the shutters came down again.

She laughed uncomfortably. '*Chuckles* is a pretty benign nickname. Are you sure?' She hid her discomfiture in action as she attached her camera to the monopod.

'It was because he used to laugh whenever they gave him a body to dispose of.'

'Oh.'

'Just be careful around him. From what I understand, he can be a little unpredictable.'

She narrowed her eyes at him. 'You're having me on.'

Krish laughed. She wished he wouldn't laugh. She'd missed that laugh.

He whipped out his phone, scrolled to an article on Google, and passed it to her. Her eyes got bigger and bigger as she read about the father of the bride. 'Shit, he spent fifteen years in prison.'

'So you'll be careful?' he said, tucking the phone into his jacket pocket.

'Well, yeah. As careful as I can be, I guess.' She'd have to make sure she didn't run her mouth off in front of Chuckles anymore. She didn't want to end up in a shallow grave for the crime of being rude.

Krish took a step away from her. 'It's nice to see you again, Francesca. You look good.' He turned and walked back to the groom's party.

She didn't want to admit that his words made her breath catch in her throat. Or that she'd clocked his empty ring finger.

## 2

Of all the weddings in all the world, why did she have to turn up at this one?

Krish ran his hands over his face, not for the first time that day. He felt like he had two jobs: the first one, photographing the event and the second one, keeping an eye on Francesca.

It was chaos.

The bland hotel ballroom echoed with the repetitive chorus of 'Rabbit', performed by a Chas and Dave tribute band. Guests hopped up and down on the dance floor with the energy of toddlers high on cake. Littered around the perimeter, the round, linen-covered tables were stained with the leftovers of the wedding breakfast. The bride and groom themselves were absent. Krish knew for a fact that they were upstairs screwing in their room again. Francesca was filming the dance floor from the outskirts, on the opposite side from him.

He had never been to a wedding where two worlds came crashing together so magnificently. On the one side there was the bride's family, who looked like extras from a biopic about the Krays. Their smart suits covered more than just muscle (he saw a cousin of the bride snorting coke off the edge of a switchblade). Larry sat at his table like a Cockney Michael Corleone, his bodyguard standing to attention at his shoulder and the shrivelled husks of once-tough old men arranged around him in a gangster tableau of the Last Supper.

On the other side, there was the groom's family, so middle class that they all probably had full ISAs, up-to-date wills, and a second home in Cornwall. His parents and relatives were huddled around their table like it was a raging bonfire, the only thing keeping them from getting eaten by wolves. Robert's mother had cried dramatically during the ceremony, at a volume that made it hard to hear the vows. Must be hard to watch the son she thought was a respectable lawyer marry into a crime family.

Thankfully, it was home time.

Krish unslung the heavy camera from around his neck and packed it into his bag, glad the wedding was over for him. On a normal day, he would have found this whole scenario hilarious, but today, it had just been exhausting, mentally and physically.

All thanks to Francesca March.

Krish closed his eyes, reliving the moment he first saw her pop out from behind the groom. His stomach muscles had clenched like he'd been punched. In the five years since they'd broken up, she'd changed...and she hadn't. The same long, dark hair. The same intelligent green eyes. She was still curvy, but also seemed more toned. And her breasts...

Both the attraction and the heartache had been immediate.

She was 'the one that got away'. Just when he'd thought they were ready to take their relationship to the next level—bam!—she'd dropped a bomb on him: she'd met another man—some bloke named Norman, for chrissakes.

It had completely blindsided him.

Up until Francesca, Krish had led a charmed life. When he wanted something, he usually got it—not with money, but with good luck, hard work, and a friendly, appealing manner. Things always seemed to happen for him. After secondary school, he'd gone to

Oxford and completed a law degree. After graduating near the top of his class, he worked as a lawyer for a couple of years, before deciding it wasn't for him. He wanted to pursue his photography hobby as a career.

Spurred on by Francesca—in fact, she was the only person in his life that told him to go for it—he'd applied for an assistant role with Connor Knight. Of course, he got it. Krish had beat out hundreds of applicants for that job, and he and Francesca went to Paris for a long weekend to celebrate. He remembered watching her sleep in the stripes of morning sunlight cast by the wooden blinds that didn't close all the way.

When it came to women, he never had a problem. He had always been the one to break things off when it wasn't going well or got boring.

Until Francesca.

Until she'd broken his heart.

Across the room, he saw her retrieving her mic pack from the father of the bride. Krish bunched his fingers as the lecherous gangster pulled her into a hug. He knew how Francesca felt about hugs from strangers, which is why he was unsurprised when she pretended to step on the gangster's foot by accident. She backed away from him, half-heartedly apologising as she went. Krish chuckled quietly. She always did know how to take care of herself.

Krish waited to ensure she got safely away from the man before zipping up his camera bag and wheeling it towards the exit.

Once outside, he sucked in a deep breath, wondering if he should say goodbye to her.

No. He should leave now. Go straight home, call Jess, and get an early night before his meeting with Connor tomorrow.

He was about to start towards the tube when Francesca appeared next to him, laden with bags. The exhaust-heavy London air swirled around them.

'That was one hell of a wedding,' she said casually.

He narrowed his eyes at her. He wondered what had happened with her and Norman. Were they still together? What had she been up to for the last five years? Was she still making documentaries?

'Fancy a drink?' he asked, surprising himself. The thought had completely skipped his frontal cortex and gone straight to his mouth.

He was even more surprised when she said, 'Yeah, sure.'

SHIT, BALLS, AND BOLLOCKS. WHAT WAS SHE DOING HERE?

The last thing Francesca wanted was a tell-all reunion. And yet here she was, surrounded by their bags at a corner table in the Bleeding Hart, watching Krish order drinks at the bar while she tore up a beermat. He smiled his wide smile at the barmaid, who was laughing with him about something. Of course she was. Everybody loved Krish.

Today had been a trial. Between the best man's grabby hands, her ex-boyfriend turning up, and the dull pain in her abdomen, this wedding had sucked beyond the usual. Larry, as it happened, had taken a shine to her and had chatted and joked with her all day like she was one of his gang. But his friendship had an edge to it. It reminded her of Pike, her childhood dog. One second he'd be licking her and begging for attention. The next, he'd try to sink his teeth into her. Larry felt a bit like that. She saw him flip when the bride's brother made an inane, but harmless, joke. One second they were laughing and then—fangs out. She was glad to escape before she'd experienced his bite.

Krish returned to the table, moving with his casual, leonine grace: the walk of a man who was confident that the world was on his side. She used to envy this quality in him, his self-belief and the faith that everything would work out. She'd love just an ounce of that.

He passed her the vodka, lime, and soda. Their fingers grazed, and her hand jerked involuntarily, spilling some drops on the table.

Unfazed, Krish sat down and removed his tie, tucking it into his camera bag. As he undid the first few buttons of his shirt, a hint of dark hair peeked out. She remembered hours spent in bed, running her hands through it.

'Cheers,' she said, lifting her drink.

'Cheers.'

They both took a sip and slipped into silence.

He cleared his throat. 'I, um, can't stay too long. I've got to call my girlfriend soon, check in.'

*Smooth*, she thought. He couldn't have crowbarred the mention of a girlfriend into the conversation any less conspicuously if he'd tried.

Francesca leaned back into the shadows and crossed her arms. So he had a serious girlfriend...that was good. Safe. Even so, she had to concentrate to keep her voice steady when she said, 'So how have you been? Are you still assisting Connor Knight?'

He sipped his beer. 'Yup. Connor's on a round-the-world trip with his wife and baby right now. Pretty much handed me his business while he's gone.'

She bit her lip and shook her head.

'What?' he asked, all innocence.

'Jammy bugger.' Their eyes met and they laughed before retreating into their drinks again. She always used to tease him about how opportunities seemed to fall into his lap.

Krish strummed his long, tapered fingers on the table. 'And you? What have you been up to? Are you still...are you still with Norman?'

Norman? That's right. She'd named her relationship-wrecking mystery lover after Norman Bates in *Psycho*. 'No, we broke up.' Her chest tightened. Another lie on the pile.

'Oh. I'm sorry,' he said in a voice that implied the opposite.

She had to move the conversation away from this line of questioning. 'So are you still torturing girlfriends with Bollywood films?'

He threw his head back and laughed, treating her to his infectious smile. 'No, I learned my lesson there.'

'What was the name of that one you made me suffer through?' She knew exactly what it was called. She'd watched it at least ten times since they'd broken up.

'*Dilwale Dulhania Le Jayenge.*'

'Or as I call it "Three Hours of My Life I'll Never Get Back."' She propped her head on her hand.

He sipped his beer. 'I'm getting the feeling you didn't like it...'

They'd had this conversation before. It was safe ground. 'The main character is a sexist pig and the girl needs to grow a pair. And I could drive a truck through the plot holes.'

'Jeez. Tell me what you really think.'

'I'd love to say that I enjoyed the cinematography...but even that was a bit ropey. Sorry.' She stirred her drink with the straw, counting on the incendiary nature of her comments to draw a response.

He threw his hands in the air. *Bingo*. 'It's an iconic Bollywood film. A classic!'

She smiled. 'Well, if it makes you feel any better, I hate *Gone with the Wind*, too.'

'So, you don't like sexist movies then?'

'Not really.'

'But your favourite film is *Moulin Rouge*. A film about a place that glorifies women for their bodies.'

'But that's not what it's *about*.' She was enjoying herself. They'd always loved bantering about movies.

'You're kidding me, right?' He leaned his elbows on the table. 'Satine is sold to the highest bidder. And speaking of plot holes, she's dying of a degenerative lung disease, but can belt out a tune right up to the time of her death?'

Playfully rolling her eyes, she said, 'You're missing the point. It's about stripping away societal labels and realising that we have more in common than not.'

'Well, so is *DDLJ*. Raj and Simran come from different back-grounds, but they're still meant to be together.'

'He's a stalker! He literally follows her to India and insinuates himself into her family's life by secretly trapping her fiancé and then freeing him. That is not normal behaviour.'

They both laughed. A little of her tension slipped away.

Stabbing pain below her abdomen caused her to stop short. *Shit.* The co-codamol was wearing off. She needed to top herself up. Suddenly she was Cinderella, and the clock was about to hit midnight.

'Um…sorry. I need to go.' She stood abruptly and started loading herself with bags. She concentrated on breathing through the pain, which made her sound like she'd just run a marathon. Probably for the best that she left anyway. Nothing good would come of this little reunion.

She saw a flash of concern in his eyes. He jumped to his feet and tried to help.

'Krish. I'm fine.' Another stab of pain. She hid it by bending over to pick up her backpack. She silently cursed. If her period was starting, she'd be in bed all day tomorrow and probably the next day as well. She couldn't afford to lose the time. Too much editing to do.

She couldn't wait for her operation, conveniently booked for October, the end of wedding season. Only a few months to go.

'Well, do you have a card or something? It'd be great to keep in touch.'

*Would it?* She wasn't sure about that, which is why she astonished herself when her hand slipped into her pocket and put her card on the table.

He picked it up. 'Your office is in Finchley Road?'

'It's cheap.'

'I don't live far from there. I bought a flat in Camden.'

'Yeah, well, maybe we could get together and exchange favourite recipes sometime.' She meant it to sound light, but it came out snarky. The pain sometimes made it hard to be civil.

Krish flinched and she dropped her gaze to the ground, guilt at her sarcasm making her skewer the inside of her lip between her teeth.

Her muscles spasmed again. Breathing hard, Francesca arranged her bags on her shoulders until she was balanced. She needed to get out of there, fast. 'Well, it's been fun,' she said before gunning for the exit.

# 3

THE SEATBELT LIGHT PINGED ON, waking Stella Price-Knight from her slumber. It took her a moment to remember where she was. Another plane. It shouldn't have been a surprise, really. She'd been on so many over the past six months. It should've been glamorous but it was hard work with a toddler in tow. Thank god they could afford business class.

She rubbed her eyes. That's right. Nairobi to London. The last leg of their round-the-world trip.

Glancing at the seating pod next to hers, she wondered where her husband, Connor, was. The sound of a giggling child made her look behind her. There. He was in the galley, wearing Grace on his chest in a patterned sling they'd been given in Rwanda. She was laughing as the flight attendant played peek-a-boo with her. Taking her turn to hide, Grace buried her red head in Connor's shoulder. He said something and the flight attendant laughed, touching his arm and leaning towards him, as though he'd said the wittiest thing in the world. Stella could imagine the smell of the woman's duty-free Chanel engulfing her poor daughter.

Rolling her eyes, Stella leaned back in her chair. She should be used to it by now, the way other women reacted to her husband, the way he reacted to them. She understood that Connor flirted with everyone: man, woman, young, or old. It was just his way. But sometimes it rankled.

A tinny voice announced, 'The pilot has turned on the fasten seatbelt sign. We are beginning our descent into London Heathrow.'

Connor appeared next to her and unwrapped Grace from the sling. 'Hey, sleepy head.'

'Hey.' Stella smiled up at him, hoping that she hadn't accidentally smudged her mascara everywhere as she slept.

Grace held out her arms and Connor handed her to Stella. She cuddled their daughter, breathing in her sweet one-year-old scent before clipping her into the infant seatbelt.

'You missed breakfast. I saved you this.' He pulled a squashed oat bar out of his back pocket and handed it to Stella. As he settled himself back into his seat, she caught an older woman across the aisle making no attempt to hide that she was ogling Connor. Her gaze shifted to Stella. The woman raised her eyebrows and nodded her head as though congratulating Stella. Connor remained oblivious.

'You remembered to book a taxi?' Stella asked.

'Yup. Krish is sorting it.' She opened her mouth to speak and he cut her off. 'Yes, I asked him to request a child seat.' He gave her his devastating half smile and a rush of heat unexpectedly bloomed under her abdomen. When would she stop having such a physical reaction to him? Never, she hoped.

Sometimes, she still couldn't believe she was married to Connor Knight. A handful of years ago, she had been a newcomer to wedding photography, and he'd been the rockstar of the industry, with a penchant for dating Scandinavian models and driving classic cars. Now he was Connor Knight: husband and father. Right now, her life was perfect.

Just as she had the thought, her imagination served up a horror story: Connor, dying horribly, falling out of a helicopter as he did aerial shots for a wedding. Her, a widow; Grace, fatherless. Mentally, she slapped herself. *Stop it, Stella.* She didn't know why, but every time she acknowledged how happy she was, her brain created some fictional tragedy to bring her back down to earth. It was really annoying.

She kissed the top of Grace's head and settled in for landing.

LONDON WAS JUST WAKING UP FOR A LAZY SUNDAY AS THE TAXI SPED towards their home in Little Venice. After the wedding, they'd sold Connor's flat to move somewhere more family-oriented. Their new five-bedroom house backed onto an immaculate communal garden, where the sound of playing children floated through the windows all day long and they could walk easily to Regent's Park and the zoo. Also, it wasn't far from Claudia, Stella's best friend, who lived in Holland Park with her husband and their twins. Connor's studio, however, remained across town, near his ex-bachelor pad in Old Street.

As they pulled up, Stella experienced an odd sense of displacement. Even though this was her home and it was familiar to her, it also wasn't. Just yesterday, she had been in Africa. Now she was on a suburban London street lined with birch trees. It felt like Little Venice had been frozen in time. Nothing had changed except the season—now midsummer—which was both disappointing and reassuring. She felt like a different person from the one that had left here six months ago. Surely, everything should have changed in her absence?

While Connor unloaded the bags, Stella carried Grace up the front steps and unlocked the door. The smell of bleach and furniture polish hit her in the face. The cleaning company had come to freshen up the place in advance of the Knights' homecoming. She walked into the hallway and slid the keyring onto an empty hook. The house was still, like a museum showcasing the living habits of 21st Century city dwellers. *And here, to the left, is a sofa set from Harrods, demonstrating a pleasing grey and yellow colour palette popular at the time.* She remembered the multiple, lengthy conversations between her and Connor about which sofa combination to purchase. Through the lens of everything she'd experienced and seen in the last six months, it seemed like such a silly thing.

Still, it was good to be home.

The door clicked closed behind her, and she swivelled to see Connor surrounded by suitcases. The thought of unpacking them made her shudder.

'Home, sweet home,' he said and walked towards her. He put his arms around them, kissing Stella's auburn head. Grace laughed and slapped his cheek with her chubby hand. Connor sniffed the air. 'I think somebody might need a change.'

'On it.' Stella grabbed the travel bag and took her daughter up the two flights of stairs to the nursery. She packaged the poop-filled nappy into a baggie and looked around for somewhere to dispose of it. Where did they keep the nappy bin? Then she remembered. They kept it in the bathroom because the plastic bin looked ugly with the decor of Grace's room. But the bathroom was at the end of the hall. What a silly place to put the bin. Post-travel Stella valued practicality over aesthetic. She'd move it back into Grace's room later.

As they came back down the stairs, the electronic ring of the doorbell reverberated through the house. Connor had disappeared along with the suitcases, so Stella answered it.

'Surprise!'

On her doorstep stood Claudia, eyes hidden behind large Italian sunglasses. Her geometrically accurate black bob had grown out. Since marrying Magnus, she'd shifted away from the sixties-style clothes she'd loved as a single woman, towards chic, patterned dresses from small French design houses. Stella thought she recognised Claudia's belted, red floral dress from a copy of *Vogue* she'd flipped through on the plane.

'How did you know we'd be home?' Stella slid Grace onto her hip and used her free arm to hug her best friend.

'At your bon voyage party, I stole your phone and approved myself for location sharing. I've been following you online since you left.'

'That's...creepy.' Stella stepped back so Claudia could step inside, carrying a jute Daylesford Organic bag.

'What if you were all kidnapped by pirates? Somebody would need to tell the police where you were.'

'Pirates?'

'Yes, fucking pirates!' Claudia clicked her tongue. 'Sorry, Gracie. I mean *effing* pirates. I read an article about some couple that were taken hostage off the coast of Somalia. It's a thing.'

'Well, we weren't on a boat, so we had about as much chance of getting taken by pirates as you do of stopping swearing.' Stella noted something else that hadn't changed: Claudia's futile attempts to reform her potty mouth. After having children, she had started making a concerted effort to clean up her language. Magnus made her put £5 in a jar every time she slipped up, which he then spent at the pub. He told Stella that he usually had enough to buy a few rounds for his friends.

'Anyway, you look amazing,' said Claudia. She made her way to the kitchen and began unpacking milk, eggs, pastries, and other cupboard essentials.

Her stomach grumbling, Stella seized a cinnamon swirl and handed half a croissant to Grace, who squirmed until Stella plopped her onto the floor.

'Hey, Claudia,' said Connor as he entered the kitchen, as though they had just seen each other yesterday. He kissed her on both cheeks. 'How's the family?'

'Drowning in Lego and barely surviving the fearless fours.'

'Ooh, pastries.' He grabbed a pain au chocolat. 'Price, I've left the suitcases in the laundry. I'm just going to pop to the studio for a quick update with Krish.'

Stella almost choked. 'What do you mean, you're going to work? We just got home. There's stuff to do.'

'I won't be long. Just a few hours.'

She sighed with exasperation. She knew that 'just a few hours' probably meant 'see you in the morning.' He'd get stuck into something, the time would slip by, and he would suddenly realise that it was almost midnight. Meanwhile, she'd be sorting through dirty clothes, dealing with the effects of long-distance travel on a toddler, and doing an on-line shop to restock their cupboards, all alone. She was annoyed, but also too tired to argue about it now.

'Fine,' she mumbled. But if he thought she was going to be doing all that laundry on her own, he had another thing coming.

'Bye, Gracie.' He kissed his pointer finger, leaned down, and placed the kiss on his daughter's nose. Her mouth covered in croissant crumbs, she smiled her gummy smile at him and said, 'Dada!'

Connor grinned like a besotted fool, and Stella's heart softened. She turned her cheek towards him, expecting a kiss of her own, but he had already left the room. *He must be really excited to see Krish*, she thought. The front door clicked closed moments later.

Grace pushed herself into a standing position and took a few tentative steps in the direction that Connor had gone. She walked a few feet and then flopped down on her bottom. 'Dada!' she called.

'Oh my god,' said Stella. 'Clauds, those were her first steps!'

'Fuck me!' said Claudia. 'Sorry, I mean, great job, Gracie!'

Both women crowded around her, and Stella picked her up for a cuddle. 'Connor is going to be gutted he missed that.'

'Let's just recreate the moment and film it. That's what iPhones were invented for.'

Stella placed her daughter on her feet and shuffled away from her while Claudia hit record. The toddler took a few steps, wobbling but determined, straight into Stella's arms. As mother and godmother praised her, Grace beamed up at them and did another first for the camera. 'Fuck!' she said proudly.

. . .

24

ONE HOUR AND MANY STEPS LATER, STELLA PUT GRACE DOWN FOR A nap and joined Claudia for coffee in the living room.

'So, how was it?' Claudia asked, pulling one bare foot onto the sofa.

'Amazing. Life-changing. It's hard to put into words. Did you see all the pictures I posted on Instagram?'

'Of course. Every. Single. One.'

'I know. I know. There were a lot. But we saw so much! And I'm trying to grow my socials.'

Claudia sipped from her mug. 'Holy shit, this is great coffee.'

'It's from Thailand. It's been pooped out by elephants.'

'That's disgusting. I don't suppose you brought any back for me?'

'No, but I *did* buy you a penis-shaped bottle opener from Bangkok.' They had a long-standing tradition of giving each other crap gifts. Stella noticed that Claudia was leaning on the wedding present she'd made them: a pillow printed with Connor and Stella's faces under the words 'Getting Hitch'. It was truly horrendous. In Grace's newborn phase, Stella had used it as a breast feeding pillow.

'Gee. Thanks. So what was your favourite part of the trip?'

'Um...gosh, there were so many places I loved. If I had to choose one...'

Claudia checked her watch.

'...I'd say Rwanda. Such a beautiful country. We met this girl in Kigali. Colette. She saw us taking pictures and approached us to talk about photography. Turns out she's extremely talented—'

'God, I'm so *jealous*. What I wouldn't give to have six months away from my life.'

Stella hid her resigned smile in her coffee mug. Claudia was obviously done hearing about the trip.

'I'm shooting all these terribly rich people now and, seriously, they do my head in. More money than sense, the lot of them. The other day, I had a client from some country ending with *'stan'* and they actually brought Kalishnikovs and swords to the shoot. For a family picture!'

With a glance at the white Cartier watch on Claudia's wrist, Stella raised an eyebrow. Since marrying into the Fiennes, Claudia had become terribly rich, too. Magnus not only worked as a wedding photographer to the Eton, Harrow, and Oxbridge set, but also managed a property portfolio that would make the Duke of Westminster green with envy. The Fiennes were old money.

Claudia drained the rest of her cup. 'When are you going back to work?'

Deflating, Stella said, 'Good question. Connor and I haven't discussed it in much detail. He seems to have assumed that I'm now full-time childcare until a spot opens up at a nursery.'

'Why don't you just get a nanny?'

Stella started shaking her head no before Claudia even finished. 'Connor prefers a nursery. He doesn't like the idea of some stranger traipsing around town with our child.'

'God forbid,' said Claudia defensively.

Remembering that her friend had a dedicated nanny for each of her boys, Stella rubbed her temple and said, 'Sorry, I didn't mean it like that.' Jet lag had made her speak without thinking, even though deep down inside, she considered having two nannies excessive. Her thoughts turned to the many mothers and children she'd seen on their trip. After travelling the world for six months and observing family life in a number of different cultures, Stella was keenly aware of her privilege even having this conversation about childcare. Furthermore, she was lucky that she actually had the choice to work or not. But after the long flight, her brain couldn't handle that discussion right now. 'I'm just tired.'

Claudia flapped her hand to dismiss the unintended slight. 'She's on a waiting list at Doodlebug Daycare, right?' Doodlebug was the top nursery in the area.

'Yes! And Bubblegum Babies, Wee Wonders, and Cuddly Cougars! But none of them can guarantee when a place will become available.'

'Didn't you put her name down when you were pregnant?'

'No, I didn't realise I had to.'

Claudia sucked in air through her teeth. 'Rookie mistake.'

'Come on! Who knew it would be harder to get a place at a good nursery than it is to become prime minister?'

'Um. *Everybody.*'

'Well, I didn't know. You could have mentioned it.' Stella nibbled her cuticles.

Putting down her mug, Claudia swiped at Stella's fingers. 'Cut that out. Haven't you kicked that habit yet? You've been relaxing for six months.'

'Relaxing? I wish,' said Stella with a huff.

Claudia narrowed her eyes. 'What's going on? Does this have something to do with that email you sent me about "wanting a change"?'

Stella bit the inside of her lip. She forgot that she'd sent that email to Claudia. She had done it when she was angry at Connor because he'd taken on another impromptu shooting assignment on what was supposed to be their family holiday. At the time, they were staying at a five-star hotel in Cape Town—a splurge for the final leg of their trip. When the hotel realised that the world's best wedding photographer was staying there, they asked him to shoot their new wedding portfolio in connection with a local luxury bridal boutique. In exchange, they'd wipe the Knights' entire bill including food, which would save them thousands—even though Stella was confident that it wasn't the money that attracted Connor to the job. She knew him well enough to know his ego was involved, and the attractive female event planner had done a good job of stoking it.

'It'll only take a day. Two at most,' he'd reasoned. But of course, it hadn't. It robbed Grace and Stella of five days with Connor while he organised and executed the shoot. Stella was stuck in the hotel entertaining Grace alone (which was when she'd started researching nurseries and signing up).

It also rankled that Connor hadn't asked Stella to be involved.

Especially since she was just as good as him. Since marrying Connor and being absorbed into his business, she'd learned a lot: posing, lighting, that ease with the camera that came only from experience. Clients could no longer tell the difference between one of her images and one of his. However, people always referred to her as 'Connor Knight's wife', rarely by her own name. When she worked a wedding with him, she never got credit for the amazing images she was shooting. Her work got subsumed into the Connor Knight brand. She'd thought about this a lot while they were travelling.

When she'd emailed Claudia, she'd been toying with an idea about moving into portraiture and working under her own brand name. While it created some problems, it also solved a few. Stella didn't like how often shooting weddings would take her away from Grace. Their daughter didn't deserve to be a wedding orphan—to have both parents working almost *every* weekend. Moving into portraiture would make it easier to have a Monday to Friday job.

Picking at some imaginary lint on her sleeve, Stella said, 'I think I'm ready to try something new.'

'What do you mean "new"? You're not going to change careers again, are you?' Four years ago, Stella had transitioned from being an advertising copywriter to wedding photographer after having an ill-fated affair with her boss.

'No, nothing like that.' She leaned back and rested the mug on her chest. 'I'm just not sure I want to carry on with weddings.'

'Ha! I told you you'd get tired of them. They're a bloody headache. What does Connor think?'

Stella frowned. 'We haven't really discussed it.'

'Why not? I'm sure he'd understand. He has Krish anyway.'

'It's just…he wants to start shooting more fashion. He keeps talking about when I eventually come back, how he can concentrate on building a new portfolio, etcetera.'

'Awkward.'

'I think...I think I want to go into portraiture. Shooting women, specifically.'

'What? Like boudoir?'

'I don't know. Maybe. I want to help women feel beautiful. When I was travelling, I saw how much having a good picture lifted some of the women I shot. Their smiles when I showed them the back of my camera...I was just posing them well in flattering light, but to them...it was magic.'

A cry on the baby monitor ripped through the room.

'Well! That's my cue to leave,' said Claudia, standing and slipping her Charlotte Olympia shoes on.

'I'll call you,' said Stella. 'Let's get dinner in the diary soon. I want to see Magnus.'

Claudia chuckled. 'Does that go for Connor, too?'

'Stop it! They get on now, don't they?' Connor and Magnus had always had a tolerate/hate relationship after years of being wedding photography rivals. Stella didn't understand it. Magnus could be a little privileged sometimes, but really he was a big teddy bear.

Suddenly serious, Claudia said, 'Stells, I think it's a good idea. You should do it.'

'Dinner?'

'The portraiture business!'

After Claudia left, Stella stood with her back to the front door and took a deep breath, thoughts racing. She was 99% sure this new course was what she wanted. In her heart and for the sake of their relationship, she knew she had to stop walking behind the famous Connor Knight. Didn't she deserve to shine, too? If she didn't do her own thing, she'd grow to resent him, and that could only be bad for their marriage.

But there were so many considerations. Was now the right time? Would Grace be okay with both of her parents running their own businesses? Would Connor understand? Would his business be okay without her? So many questions skittered around in her head, each new one appearing on the tail of the last.

As her mother used to say, *'Non si può avere la botte piena e la moglie ubriaca'*, which meant 'You can't have a barrel full of wine and a drunk wife at the same time.' Something would have to give.

She climbed the stairs towards Grace's room, hoping a solution would come to her soon.

## 4

KRISH'S FEET struck the pavement at a regular 140 beats per minute, techno pounding in his ears. The afternoon sun heated his skin, and he could feel hard-earned sweat soaking through his athletic vest.

The riverside path at the top of Battersea Park was teeming with the usual Sunday afternoon crowd: other runners, rollerbladers, kids learning to cycle, dogs lolloping, and a lot of prams. Krish needed to keep part of his brain focused on the assault course of people in front of him to avoid colliding with anyone. The other part flitted between the two subjects most on his mind: Francesca and Connor.

That morning, he'd met Connor at his studio. They'd had lunch at a local café while Connor regaled Krish with all the stories from his trip. It sounded amazing. The pictures on Connor's phone were breathtaking enough; Krish could just imagine the ones Connor had on his proper camera. By the end, Krish could feel his own feet itching to travel far-off lands.

He hadn't realised how much he'd missed Connor. He looked good. Connor always looked good, but now he had a deep tan, and his dark hair had grown longer. He could probably put it into a ponytail. He had the relaxed appearance of someone who had just come back from a six-month holiday.

But his energy told a different story. It was anything but relaxed; he wanted to get back to work. After Krish had given him an update on each client and on upcoming weddings, Connor had launched into a speech about his big plans. While Stella and Krish handled the main chunk of the wedding work, Connor wanted to branch out into fashion and advertising. All the soul-searching he'd done on the trip showed him that he was ready to make the next leap in his career.

Krish didn't have the heart to reveal that so was he.

He didn't want to disappoint Connor, but he'd been with him for over five years. It was time for Krish to start his own business. He'd even found the perfect office space close to his flat in an artsy incubator hub.

A small dog unexpectedly lurched into Krish's path and he leapt over it. Another techno song thumped through his headphones.

And then there was Francesca.

He wished that she'd remained in his past, even though part of him was glad that he'd run into her, confirming that she was alive and well. She'd disappeared from his life so suddenly after they broke up. Poof! Like they hadn't dated for six months.

Getting over her had taken a long time, even with working for Connor to distract him. He remembered the pile of self-help books about how to survive bad break-ups stacked on his coffee table. His sister Ankita nicknamed him Miss Havisham, insinuating that he'd spend his whole life hung up on Francesca if he didn't snap out of it. She told him that he needed to get 'under someone to get over someone' which was the last thing he wanted to do. Eventually, he realised that the books only made him feel worse with their contradicting advice.

He packed them up and left them at a charity shop. He moved on.

And he wanted to remain 'moved on'. Once upon a time, Francesca had been the woman he thought he might marry, the woman he'd start a family with. Then Norman came on the scene.

Fucking Norman. Who named their kid Norman these days, anyway?

Seeing her yesterday had been bittersweet. They'd fallen right back into their easy banter, talking about their favourite topic: films. It had felt like old times...until she ran out of the pub as if the fire alarm had gone off.

And that was why he couldn't shake the thought that something was wrong. As she'd gathered her kit, he'd seen a fleeting grimace of pain on her face. He didn't want to care, but he was worried about her.

Damn it.

Krish shook his head, trying to dislodge the concern that was forming.

His pace slowed and he came to a complete stop, checking his stats on his watch while he waited. Jess should be finished soon. They'd organised to regroup at Cleopatra's Needle after they each completed their distance targets.

Up ahead, a family of four caught his eye. They clutched ice cream cones in their hands, laughing as the heat made them drip, racing to lick them up. They reminded him of his own family: white mother, Indian father, brother and sister. He watched the sister bossing her younger brother around and getting frustrated when he ignored her—also like his family. Krish smiled.

A hand clapped him on the back and he jumped. He popped the headphones out of his ears as Jess appeared in front of him, breathing heavily.

'Just me!' she huffed between exhales and inhales. She flashed her dazzling smile, perfect teeth. It helped that her dad was a dentist. 'Did you set a new personal best? Looked like you were hitting a good pace.'

'Not really. Lost in thought.' He gave her his water bottle.

She took a long sip and handed it back. 'Connor?'

'Yeah.' She didn't need to know about Francesca. It didn't mean anything. Jess had been the one to help him piece his heart back together again. Jess was his future.

She flopped forwards and touched her toes, the tip of her long, blonde plait brushing the pavement. 'Maybe you're holding back because you don't really want to leave. Are you sure you need to do this? It pays well...the work is interesting...'

Pressing his lips together, he mentally flicked away a blossom of irritation. He wished she wouldn't question his plans every time he brought them up. Her aversion to risk came from growing up as an only child with kind, but overprotective parents. However, he also knew her heart was in the right place. She just wanted a stable, secure future for them.

And that was exactly what he would deliver. In his mind, this new path wasn't risky at all.

Krish kicked his foot towards his bottom and caught it with his hand, stretching his quads. 'No, I'm confident this will work out. And I'm ready for a change.' Connor had taught him everything he knew. Despite the fact that he was only ten years older than Krish, he thought of Connor as more than a boss, or even a friend. He was a mentor and father figure. 'I just don't want to appear ungrateful.'

He moved to the wall, lifted his leg and perched it on top. As he stretched his hamstrings, Jess copied him.

'Don't forget you did him a huge favour, watching his business while he had a six-month holiday.'

'Yeah, but I kept the money from all the jobs I shot for him—'

'—Minus twenty-five percent.'

'It's a finder's fee. I didn't mind paying it.'

'My point is, he couldn't have done it without you, so don't act like it's all one-sided, hon. You have a rainbow inside of you, waiting to shine.' She poked him in the chest over his heart.

Krish smiled. The primary school teacher in Jess had an optimistic way of speaking that often involved references to rainbows, unicorns, and glitter.

He threw a sweaty arm over her shoulder and planted a kiss on her forehead. Things were so easy with Jess. That's what all his married friends said was the key difference between the ones they married and the ones they didn't. The relationships were just easier. No games. No drama. Goals in line. Krish remembered having The Conversation with Jess about whether she wanted kids on their third or fourth date. (The answer was yes). It just came up naturally as they were chatting. No big deal.

Staring out at a boat bobbing along on the Thames, he thought about Connor and Stella. Their relationship hadn't been easy. They both fought against their obvious attraction from day one, when they met at the BAPP convention. Krish chuckled as he remembered the wedding they shot together in Italy. Connor and Stella slept together and then tried to hide it, but Krish totally knew what was going on. Before Stella, Connor had strong opinions on marriage and how it wasn't for him. Having met Connor's father, Armstrong, who never met a female he didn't hit on, he could see where Connor got his views. But then Connor met the right person, and even though the road to love had been rocky (if entertaining to watch from Krish's front row seat), they were now happily married with the cutest baby girl. It had made him want to find love, too.

'Race you back?' Jess bit her lip and winked at him suggestively.

He gave her a light, competitive slap on her bottom, and they took off jogging in the direction of her flat on Battersea Hill. As they hit a steady stride, Krish felt a vibration in his pocket. 'Wait a sec,' he called to her as he pulled up short and took out his phone. Connor's name illuminated the screen. 'Sorry, I've got to take this.' He popped his headphones in before answering: 'Hello?'

STELLA LISTENED AS CONNOR TALKED TO KRISH. THEY HADN'T EVEN been back a full day, and he was already scheduling shoots. And not just *any* shoot. A shoot with Valentina Vavilvek.

'Next Friday, yeah. Can you assist?' He sat at the kitchen table, laptop open. Grace was asleep again upstairs, her body clock skewed by travel. Stella worried they'd both be up all night again.

'Great. At her Mayfair house, yup. Super. I'll book her in and send you the details.'

He hung up.

Stella stood at the counter, aggressively cutting peppers with a sharp knife. 'That was fast.'

'Hmmm?' She could tell he wasn't really listening as he typed an email.

'How did she even know you were back? Is she spying on you?' Stella yawned as she brought the knife down, almost slicing her finger open. Even irritation couldn't dull her exhaustion.

'Um, I think she saw it on my Instagram or something.'

Stella tossed the peppers into the wok and they sizzled noisily in the oil.

'So what did she get this time? A new car? Another boob job? Botox?' Valentina was addicted to boudoir shoots with Connor. She had one every few months, every time she got a new toy or new surgery. Connor probably knew Valentina's body better than he knew Stella's.

Connor continued typing. 'A diamond necklace from Tiffanys, I believe.'

'Hmmm.' She moved onto the broccoli, tearing off the florets with surprising force. 'Will her husband be there?'

'I try not to think too hard about where her husband is.'

Another reason that Stella didn't like Connor being involved with the Vavilveks: her husband, Asbjorn, was a money launderer for the Scandinavian elite. Valentina had let it slip during one of her shoots with Connor. Apparently, he was semi-retired, which didn't make Stella feel better in the slightest. She didn't like the idea of where their money came from. She said as much.

Connor sounded so convincing when he replied, 'I know, but one shoot with her will pay for an entire year of school for Grace.'

'Oh? Have we decided that she's going to an independent school then?' This was an area where Connor and Stella had differing views. As the child of a diplomat, Connor had attended a string of private schools around the world. He thought paying for education would open more doors for his daughter and he wanted only the best. Stella, however, went to state schools right up until university and had an amazing education. She believed that they should keep Grace in the state system. Of course, their daughter was only one. They didn't need to come to any decisions for a while.

Connor ignored her question as he finished typing and closed his computer. He got up from the stool and walked around the island, slipping his arms around Stella from behind and nuzzling her neck. Stella stood stiff, stirring the vegetables with added vigour. He couldn't just seduce his way out of trouble.

But then he slipped his hand into her underwear and she drew in a sharp breath. Her back softened; her head leaned onto his shoulder. Suddenly she didn't feel tired at all.

Deep down she knew that he was playing her, wielding their fierce attraction to diffuse a tense situation. After two years of marriage and two years together before that, they enjoyed a well-honed sex-life. They both found that any problems they had seemed to dwindle when viewed through a post-coital haze.

His finger slid inside her and she groaned. Their chat about Valentina could wait.

'How long has Grace been sleeping?' he whispered in her ear.

'About thirty minutes...' She reached back and grabbed a tuft of his newly shoulder-length hair. Hopefully he wouldn't cut it now that they were back. It was so incredibly sexy.

He removed his hands from her pants and flipped her around in his arms. 'That should give us just enough time...'

'To install the stair gate? Needs to be done.' She smiled and bit her lip coyly.

'Later. I had something else in mind.' He turned off the hob and pulled her towards the sofa.

The stair gate would have to wait.

## 5

KRISH'S FINGER hovered over the buzzer. *March Films* was written in Sharpie on top of the plastic. He looked up at the building, a seventies-style office block, concrete and glass with smudged windows, each bisected horizontally by off-white slatted blinds in various states of disarray: some straight, some on angles, most with bent or missing slats. It was a far cry from Connor's luxury studio in Islington.

He shouldn't be here. Francesca probably wouldn't welcome the surprise. But he'd been in the area, dropping off a camera for repair. The curiosity to see where she worked had wormed its way into his thoughts to the point where he had to either act or go for a long, long run. He chose action.

Besides, he was worried about her. She'd left the bar so suddenly last Saturday. He wanted to check everything was okay.

Taking a deep breath, he pressed the bell and waited. No reply. Maybe she wasn't in. He took out his phone and dialled the number on her card. It hadn't changed in five years. Neither had his. He wondered whether she still had his number in her phone or if she'd deleted it.

'This is Francesca March from March Films...'

He listened to the entire message, but hung up before the beep.

Stepping towards the front door, he realised it wasn't properly closed. Somebody had left it on the latch. Not very safe. Glancing left and right, he tugged the door open and walked through.

Her office, number 105, was on the first floor. From somewhere on the upper floors, heavy metal music reverberated through the halls. Krish climbed the stairs, ignoring the tangled odour of urine, mould, and bleach. He passed an older woman on her way down, dressed in an ill-fitting grey suit and clutching her briefcase like she thought Krish might relieve her of it. Standing aside, he smiled and nodded, pressing his tall frame into the corner of the landing, trying to be unthreatening. She clopped to the bottom of the stairs and rushed out of the building. He sighed.

The hallway made him think of a deserted secondary school with the magnolia-painted breeze blocks, flickering fluorescent lighting, and occasional noticeboards. Somebody had even written a cheery 'Fuck You' on one of them. Charming.

Francesca's office was at the end of the hall, behind a grey fire door covered in locks. The padlocks at the top and bottom were missing and he felt his pulse pick up. Maybe she was in after all.

He knocked.

From the other side, he heard a chair scraping against the floor and items being knocked over. 'Who is it?' Francesca's voice shouted.

'It's Krish!'

The muffled curse that followed confirmed that perhaps this had been a bad idea.

Metal scratched metal as she unlocked the door. With sudden force, it swung open, a hand reached out, grabbed Krish's sleeve, and pulled him into the room. Francesca shut the door behind him and reengaged the locks.

It took a moment for Krish's eyes to adjust. A bank of three large video screens offered the room's only illumination, sunlight blocked by thick black curtains hanging over the windows. In contrast to the hallway, the room smelled strongly of pine, as though Francesca had an economy box of air fresheners somewhere and had opened them all at once.

But Krish's gaze went straight to Francesca, who had a cricket bat over one shoulder and a cross look on her face. Even in the blue light of the screens, he could see the dark circles under her eyes.

'What the bloody hell are you doing here?' Her words held fire, but the delivery sounded flat.

'Jesus, Francesca, you look terrible.' She wore grey tracksuit bottoms and a white tank top. Her arms were bare, showing off a surprising amount of muscular definition. When they'd dated, she hadn't been much of a gym person, but maybe that had changed.

'Well, if I'd known you were coming, I would have hired a make-up artist. Gotten a manicure.'

'You know what I mean. When's the last time you slept?' He kicked an empty can of Red Bull aside.

'Tuesday?'

It was Thursday.

She shuffled back to her desk, sank into the chair, and propped the bat against the leg of the table.

On the middle screen, a frozen close up of a laughing bride watched on.

'Sounds healthy,' he observed.

Francesca snorted. 'No time for healthy. Deadlines.' She jutted her chin towards the screens. Grasping the mouse, she clicked the play button. The sound of applause and laughter filled the room for a moment before she hit pause again and nudged a slider to the right. She played the clip again, nodded, and moved on to the next clip.

Krish sighed. This was not going well. 'I brought you coffee and a donut.'

'Thanks. But I don't eat sugary snacks.'

'Oh. Since when?'

'Since none of your business.' She swivelled her chair towards him. 'I'll take the coffee though.'

He handed her the cup.

'Ugh. Starbucks. The local cafe around the corner is so much better.'

'You're welcome.'

She rolled her eyes and half-smiled. Showing gratitude had never been her strong point.

On the walls, there were multiple white boards, covered in to-do lists and dates. The one marked *Weddings* at the top had ten last names in a column. In a second column with the heading *Due*, was a list of dates—all in the past. Only two had lines through them, marking them complete. 'So this is where you work?'

'It's in budget.'

'Is it safe?'

She shrugged and took a sip of her coffee.

With surprise, he noticed a kitten-themed calendar stuck to the wall. Not the animal he'd immediately associate with her, but okay. He saw she had three weddings scheduled this month. In the bottom corners of most of the squares, she had scribbled letters in Sharpie: some had a C, some a P, and others a red B. He wondered what they meant. 'Why don't you work from home?'

'Flat's too small.'

Krish nodded his head. 'You seem pretty busy. That's good.'

'I know I'm supposed to say something twee like "Can't complain", but I actually can. I have too many weddings and no time to work on other projects.'

'Are you charging enough?'

She shook her head and held up her hand. 'Stop right there. I don't need you to fix this for me. It's my problem.'

'Come on, Francesca. I've been working for Connor Knight for the past five years. I've learnt a fair share about business and pricing in that time.'

'What about you? What's your big plan? I know you'll have one.'

'Me?' He could tell she was changing the subject on purpose. He'd circle back later. 'It's time for me to go off on my own. My *plan* is to focus on Indian weddings. Good money. And they're exciting. Colourful.' As usual when he thought about his plan, it was accompanied by a sinking feeling in his stomach. He wasn't looking forward to the conversation he needed to have with Connor tomorrow after the Valentina Vavilvek shoot.

Silence wrapped itself around them. He had definitely been right: something was wrong. She had always been a hard worker—often cancelling dates last minute due to her old job—but this was taking things to a whole new level. He knew that she wouldn't appreciate it if he pried. She'd always been the sort of person who didn't like to talk about herself or accept help from others. When they'd been dating, it had taken a while to get her to open up to him about her upbringing: her Olympian parents and their high expectations of her —their disappointment when she hadn't turned out to be an amazing athlete like her older sister and two brothers.

Maybe he could get her to talk, if he asked the right questions.

He opened his mouth.

And she grabbed her waste bin and vomited.

'Oh my god.' Krish dropped his bag and stepped towards her, holding her dark hair with one hand and rubbing her back with the other. He could feel the hard vertebrae of her spine. His hand continued to move back and forth, rising and falling with the rapid movement of her lungs.

For a moment, she seemed to relax under his touch. Her shoulders went limp and her head fell forward. But it only lasted a few seconds.

Her body stiffened. She spit into the basket and let it fall back to the floor, wiping her mouth with a crumpled napkin. 'Sorry about that. Coffee on an empty stomach.'

'This is ridiculous, Francesca.'

She stood up, breaking the contact. Grabbing the bin, she walked to the door and placed it in the hallway outside.

Krish regarded her with concern. 'You're killing yourself. Don't you have an assistant? Anybody to help?'

'Nobody would do as good a job as me.'

'You'd be surprised.' He remembered when he'd first started working for Connor. It took a few months to get down all the processes and learn how to do things exactly how Connor wanted them done, but after that, Krish had been his right-hand man. 'You just need to find the right person.'

'I can't afford to pay an assistant.'

Falling back into her chair, Francesca propped her head up on her hand. He could tell she was trembling, but trying to hide it. Krish fought the urge to hug her, the way he might have back when they were dating. He wondered if it had anything to do with her period pains. He remembered that she used to get them badly, much worse than his mother or sister ever had.

She exuded exhaustion. It made him tired just watching her. She was pushing herself too hard and, from the whiteboard covered in financial information, not charging nearly enough for her talent and time.

It took him a moment to realise she had actually fallen asleep. Her head tipped off her hand and she jerked awake.

'Sorry. What did you say?' As though she hadn't just passed out in front of him.

'Come work for me. I'm looking for somebody to run the video side of my business.' The words were out of his mouth before his brain could catch up.

What had he just said? What was it about Francesca March that made him act irrationally? He crossed his arms over his chest to stop himself from slapping his own face. The air in the room stilled as though the very molecules awaited her answer.

She blinked. And blinked again. 'Are you insane?' she finally asked, incredulity dripping from her voice. 'Have you actually lost your mind?' Her face paled, and she looked like she might be sick again.

'I know. Sorry. I don't know where that came from.' He toed a discarded food container on the floor. His skin itched with embarrassment. He had been so overwhelmed by the need to help that he'd bleated out the first thing that came to mind.

'Well, it was a pretty shit idea. Let's be honest, you don't even know me anymore.'

Krish flinched. *I'm not sure I ever did,* he thought sadly. The girl he'd thought she was wouldn't have left him for some guy named Norman.

It had been a mistake to come here. Francesca had stirred up a host of emotions he'd happily been keeping in a closed jar. Now, the memories were pushing him off-kilter. Five years was a long time, and both of them had surely evolved into different people with different lives. He knew nothing about hers, and she knew nothing about his. Best keep it that way.

'Okay...well...I've got to go. But, Francesca...do call me if you ever need help. I still care for you.'

The words slipped out of his mouth and he waited for regret to hit him, but it never did. He'd simply spoken the truth. He would always have feelings for her, want the best for her, even though they'd never be together.

With a sad smile, he walked towards the door and pulled it open. Looking back at her one last time, he realised he probably wouldn't see her again. His heart beat faster. 'Here's looking at you, kid,' he said, before he left.

LATER THAT EVENING, FRANCESCA LAY ON HER BED IN THE STUDIO apartment where she'd been living for the past couple of years. She could cover the entire width in fifteen paces and the depth in ten, but it was her oasis: a place where she didn't have to hide her pain or do anything except sleep and relax. She consciously chose to separate her office from her home. The extra cost was worth it; besides, her office was only a couple blocks away. Only 823 steps. Keeping them separate meant she could shut off.

The room was not overly fussy. The walls were a warm off-white;

the bedspread, a clean grey; the rug, a natural sisal. She would have loved to liven up the room with some plants, but she would just kill them. Instead, she had a cactus collection on top of a chest of drawers next to the window. Each cactus had a name. Freddy. Hannibal. Voldemort. And Hans Gruber.

A sharp pain clenched her uterus and she pressed her hot water bottle into the skin directly on top, letting the heat go to battle for her. Her body cried out for sleep after so much time in the office, but her mind wasn't giving her the option. It fizzled with regret.

'I still care for you.'

Krish's words replayed over and over in her head. He'd always been so much better about verbalising his feelings than she was. The echo of his touch on her back rolled through her, connecting with memories of other times he'd stroked his fingers down her spine.

Why had she been so rude to him? He'd only been trying to help. He had always been the kind of person who hated to see others suffering, and suffering she was. She must have seemed pathetic. Aside from the lack of sleep, her cramps and nausea had been intense all week. Her period started two days ago. Usually, she'd spend this time in bed, but her workload left her no choice but to soldier through. While handling the pain, her ability to talk politely with other humans suffered. Krish had walked straight into a perfect storm.

She must have looked appalling for him to have offered her a job. A bitter groan escaped her lips. She didn't want his pity.

Working with him—or anyone—wasn't an option. She needed as much flexibility as she could get in her career. Self-employment was the best choice for a woman with her issues. The thought of co-workers watching the clock to monitor her time keeping...she shivered.

Francesca had been an employee in the past. She knew the drill: at first, her employer would be sympathetic when she called in sick because of the pain. Then, as time wore on and it happened more than a few times per month, the sympathy would diminish. Having ailments that people couldn't see stretched compassion to its limits. Eventually, Francesca would quit because she couldn't stand the side-long looks and snarky comments.

*Fuck them all.*

As things were, she could set her own hours. Aside from the three weddings she'd take on per month, the only other time she crawled out of her office cave was to meet couples who wanted to book her—even then she tried to do as many of those meetings online as she could. On the wedding days themselves, it was always a game of chance as to whether she was in pain or not. Some days she won; some days she lost. But on every day, she kept moving forward.

If she worked with Krish, he'd end up judging her, too. He'd figure out pretty quickly that something was wrong with her. At first, he might just think she was lazy. Then he would ask questions and, eventually, he'd realise why she ran away all those years ago. She imagined his face as he discovered the extent of her brokenness, her lies. First, the anger. Next, the pity. Then, the relief as he walked away.

Would he understand that she'd done it for his own good? To save them both the trauma?

Probably not. She moaned with despair.

Of course, there was also the fact that she'd want to rip his clothes off all the time. Hard to get work done when fantasising about screwing your business partner on the computer desk.

A faint scratching sound caught her attention. She glanced towards her kitchenette and the sagging black bin bag in the corner. She swore. By sleeping in the office last night, she'd missed the rubbish collection, which included the compost bin under the sink. The scratching noise repeated.

*Shit balls.*

She had already suffered through one rat infestation six months earlier, which had required a costly call-out from an ineffective pest control company. The various poisons and traps they had set remained uneaten and unsprung. Thankfully, the rodents had eventually moved on of their own volition.

Tomorrow, she'd take the rubbish to work with her and dispose of it there.

Another pain ripped through her middle. She yelled out and punched the pillow next to her before slumping back onto the bed. Sometimes anger was the best medicine.

Suddenly loud music began pumping downstairs.

'Fucking great. It's Bollywood night.'

When she originally rented this flat, the space below had been gloriously empty. Then, last year, a dance company had moved in and quickly ruined her life. She could handle Ballet Mondays, Tap Tuesdays, and Pilates Wednesdays. But it was Bollywood Thursdays, Flamenco Fridays, and Contemporary Dance Saturdays that drove her up a wall.

They called her 'That Woman.'

'That Woman is here to complain again,' said the receptionist into the phone whenever Francesca could be arsed to drag herself downstairs to tell them to turn it down. She'd also lodged a complaint with the landlord. Apparently, the dance studio needed to put in sound proofing. The dance studio argued that was the landlord's responsibility.

She slumped back onto the sofa. She didn't have the energy to crawl out of bed, much less have a fight with anyone. Her eyes wandered towards her collection of Hindi movies neatly stacked under her wall-mounted television. After her break-up with Krish, she had become a secret fan of Bollywood films, although she'd never admit that to him. Watching them made her feel they still had a tenuous connection. On Friday nights, she usually curled up on the sofa and put one on. She'd pour herself a vodka and tonic to unwind and create a game out of it, taking a sip whenever someone overacted, there was a big dance number, bad CGI, random product placement, or a longing look that lasted for more than five seconds. She rarely made it to the end of the film.

Her stomach grumbled, this time with hunger rather than pain. She realised she hadn't eaten anything nutritious in three days. Usually she was so careful about what she ate, as it affected her symptoms. But she was only human, and sometimes she fell off the wagon.

Francesca pushed herself off the bed and padded to the kitchen. Five steps, each one causing pressure in her abdomen. Peering inside the fridge, the first thing she found was a bowl of pesto gnocchi topped with mould, so she opened the cupboard door where the compost bin lived.

And came face to face with a large rat.

Its whiskers twitched. It had a small, white diamond in the middle of its forehead, and it stared at her with its black, glass-bead eyes, as though asking, 'You got a problem?'

She closed the door. *Great.* Another bill she couldn't afford. She added *Call Pest Control* to her mental to do list, right above the other twenty million line items.

'Are you charging enough?' Krish had asked her. With great annoyance, she acknowledged that the answer was probably 'no'.

She really hated when he was right.

## 6

KRISH HELD THE REFLECTOR, bouncing light onto Valentina Vavilvek's naked body.

She posed next to the bed, her back pressed up against one of the four carved columns that held up the gold satin-swathed canopy. The whole house looked like King Louis XIV had thrown up in it. All gilded woodwork, gold soft furnishings, gold statues.

Valentina lifted her chin to show off the sparkling diamond necklace at her throat. The shimmer that the make-up artist had rubbed into her skin made her glow like an idol in the light. A long blonde braid hung over her bare shoulder, her pouty, Botoxed lips parted slightly, and she looked towards Connor's lens like she wanted to mount the camera. Or the man behind it.

'That's great. Hold it there,' said Connor. His shutter clicked several times.

Krish stared at a golden angel clinging to the side of a swept mirror across the room. Today was the day. Today, he'd have the conversation with Connor, insist that it was time he branched out on his own. He sent a silent request to the angel for strength.

'Krish?'

He snapped out of his thoughts to find Connor looking at him.

'Sorry, Boss. What did you say?'

'Tilt the reflector so we get some light under her chin.'

Krish readjusted and sunk back into his own thoughts. Yesterday afternoon, after he'd seen Francesca, Krish had signed the contract for his new office space in Camden. No backing out now.

'Chin down just a touch, Valentina. Now bring your hand to your throat,' said Connor. Her metallic-painted nails scratched against the necklace. Click click went the camera, and he stood up. 'That's a wrap. Great job, Valentina.'

Letting the reflector drop, Krish relaxed his arms. His pulse had been racing since they'd started this job at 8AM. How would Connor take the news? Krish respected his boss and mentor so much, the idea that they'd part angry over this made his stomach hurt. But it had to be done. He needed to see what he could accomplish on his own. The time had come.

Valentina's assistant appeared with a silk robe for her, so short that it was almost a shirt. He supposed it didn't really matter. They'd all been looking at her naked for hours now.

'Darling!' she said to Connor as she tied a knot at her waist. 'That was amazing. You must never go away again. Six months is too long for me to go without you.'

'Always a pleasure, Valentina.' Connor handed his camera to Krish and cracked his neck left and right. Out of the corner of his eye, Krish saw Valentina reach up and tuck a lock of hair behind Connor's ear, a very intimate gesture. Krish knew Connor didn't like it when female clients got handsy with him. That's why part of Krish's job was to be present on shoots. A sort of chaperone.

'I love this new hair on you.' She trailed her nails over his cheek. 'Come. I need your advice on where to hang something. It's a Van Gogh.' Reaching down, she took Connor's hand and pulled him after her.

Connor widened his eyes at Krish as though saying *save me*.

Using hand signals they'd developed over the years, Krish asked if Connor wanted him to follow, but the sound of a crash made him turn before he could see Connor's reply. The make-up artist had knocked over one of his light stands. By the time Krish had made sure the light wasn't broken, Connor and Valentina had disappeared.

He followed the direction they'd gone, but couldn't see them. He tried a couple doors. All locked.

Throwing up his hands in capitulation, Krish returned to packing up their kit and his swirling thoughts. The impending chat wasn't the only thing on Krish's mind. He couldn't stop thinking about Francesca and what a sorry state she'd been in yesterday.

She did not look well. He couldn't shake the suspicion that something was wrong with her. Not a little thing, but a big thing. He didn't want to speculate on what it was; after typing nausea into Google as a symptom and being confronted with a terrifying list of possibilities, he decided not to tread that road.

Unfortunately, thinking about her in any way led him down an assortment of other wormholes. Heartache, grief, anger...the memory of the day she left him sat like a black hole on his personal timeline, sucking in all the good events around it and leaving only the break-up. Shortly after, he'd started working for Connor and threw himself into that as a form of therapy.

He shook his head to dispel the memories, realising that he had been staring into space again. He zipped up the camera case and got to work dismantling the lights. Thinking like that wasn't good for his mental health.

Besides, he had found Jess. Dependable, beautiful Jess. They shared the same values, never argued, and both saw two kids and a dog in their future. They didn't exactly have the same hobbies—Jess had a love of crafting that he didn't share, and some of the teddy bears in her extensive collection freaked him out in a Chucky sort of way. But aside from that, his mother and father approved of her. His sister adored her (and had actually introduced them). Jess was the full package.

And Krish loved her.

As long as he had Jess to tether him, he could handle being a friend to Francesca, even though he doubted he'd see her again—which was a good thing, really. Since running into her at the wedding, the movie of their relationship had been on a constant loop in his head. The fiery sex. Their intense connection. The surprise ending.

He just wished he didn't feel this need to take care of her. Why did her happiness matter to him? He sighed as he flattened a lighting stand. It was all academic. She wasn't going to be working with him (thankfully), so none of this postulating mattered. He wasn't her boyfriend; he wasn't even her *friend*. Francesca would have to take care of Francesca.

She was a stranger to him now.

Why did that thought make him so sad?

IT WAS TWO O'CLOCK BY THE TIME THEY WERE PACKED AND HEADING back to the studio. Staring out of the van window, Krish tried to work up the courage to say the words: 'I want to start my own business.' It didn't help that, every time he imagined how this conversation might go, it ended with Connor saying good riddance and breaking all communication, taking Stella and Grace with him. Krish would miss them, too.

He licked his lips for the hundredth time. Water. That's what he needed. He searched his bag for his bottle and took a long, deep drink. A sliver of liquid snaked down the wrong pipe and he spluttered, clamping his jaw closed so he didn't spit all over the car.

'You all right?' asked Connor, glancing over quickly before returning his gaze to the road.

'Fine, fine.' He noticed a red mark on his boss's collar. 'Hey, you've got some lipstick...'

'Where?' Connor flicked down the visor and located the offending mark. 'Shit. Good spot. Stella already hates Valentina. This would be the last thing I need.'

For a moment, Krish wondered how that lipstick had gotten

there. Had anything happened between Connor and Valentina when they went out of the room? Surely not. Even though in the past, Connor had dated a lot of Scandinavian models—including Valentina's friend, Galina—all of that was pre-Stella. Connor would never cheat on his wife.

They were the epitome of couple goals.

'God, yeah,' said Krish, just to say something. *I want to start my own business.* All he had to do was open his mouth and let the words pour out. Should he do it now?

What about...now?

.........................Now?

The grey London pavements sped past. Why couldn't he just say it? His tongue sat like a potato in his mouth. The muscles that controlled his lips twitched. He started drumming his hands on his legs.

Connor stopped at a red light. 'That woman is exhausting.'

'Who?'

'Valentina.'

'Oh, yeah. Yeah.'

'But she's one of my highest spending portrait clients, so...' The light changed and he accelerated. 'Actually, she's offered to help me get some tear sheets for my new portfolio. Her best friend is a picture editor at *Vogue* Scandinavia. How do you feel about shooting in Stockholm?'

Krish offered a wan smile. 'Sounds great.' One of the perks of being Connor's assistant was the world travel. He would miss that. They'd been to every continent and every European country. There'd been South Africa, the Maldives, New York...the list was long.

'So what are you up to tonight?'

Squeezing his knees before crossing and uncrossing his arms, Krish said, 'Nothing much. Just going to Jess's flat. Watch a movie while she knits something.' She would ask if he'd told Connor. If he failed, she'd give him that pitying look that all teachers mastered when a student failed at something—even though he knew she wasn't 100% behind his decision to leave. She came from a family where stability was king. Her mother had worked at the same accountancy firm her whole life, and her father, who had opened his dentistry practice in 1980, would probably die while performing a root canal.

Connor put on the indicator and turned right. 'I'd rather be doing that. Stella's invited Claudia and Magnus over for dinner.'

'I thought you and Magnus got on now.'

'We do, we do. But sometimes he can be a little arrogant.'

Pursing his lips, Krish kept himself from pointing out that was the pot calling the kettle black. He admired and loved Connor, but humility wasn't one of his strong points.

Krish sucked in a deep breath. He needed to step off the cliff and take the plunge. He opened his mouth.

'So I take it things are still going well with you and Jess?' asked Connor.

'Yeah, good. Great.' Krish tipped his head back against his seat and banged it a few times. Why couldn't he just say it?

'Is she "The One"?'

Krish could hear the air quotes implied in Connor's tone. Despite his happily-ever-after with Stella, he still derided the idea of soul mates and the idea of there being one person for everybody.

'I think so.' Krish didn't mention the ring tucked in the back of his sock drawer. That would start a whole other discussion that he didn't want to get into right now. *Focus, Krish, focus.* They passed another set of lights. The studio was only a few streets away. It was now or never. Krish's heart beat even faster as he shifted in his seat. *C'mon, you coward. You can do this.* He scratched his ear. The words built in his mouth and he cleared his throat.

'Connor—'

A loud ringing in his pocket sliced through the air, severing Krish's momentary bravado. He sighed and reached for his phone.

Francesca's name unexpectedly flashed up onto the screen. He immediately tapped the green button. 'Hello?'

'Who's this?' she asked with a strange catch in her voice.

'It's Krish.'

'Shit! I meant to call my sister.'

He sat up. The panic in her tone was like a bucket of ice water over his head. All thoughts of talking to Connor fled. 'Tell me what's wrong, Francesca.'

'My office. It's a m-mess. I've been burgled.'

## 7

AFTER THE POLICE left with a lukewarm promise to inform her if they found anything, Francesca surveyed the damage. Her lighting stands, which had obviously been deemed too unwieldy to steal, lay scattered on the floor. Her white boards had been ripped from the wall, as though the thieves expected safes to be hidden behind them. They'd broken one of her editing screens, but left the other two. Oddly, her expensive camera equipment lay untouched in the corner.

The only things they'd actually taken were her latest back-up drives. Odd. Thankfully, another tenant had disturbed them by shouting that she'd already called the cops.

Francesca dropped her head into her hands. All the footage from the gangster wedding was on those drives and *only* those drives. She hadn't yet had time to copy the files over to her set of off-site back-ups, which lived under her bed. The only other place that footage had been was on her memory cards...and she had wiped those already in preparation for her job that weekend. She would have to take them to a specialist company to see if they could recover anything. An expensive exercise that would cost money she didn't have.

'Bollocking bollocks,' she intoned as she rubbed at her face. Just what she needed, especially on top of the pest control bill at home.

She heard footsteps in the hallway and picked up her cricket bat, heart thumping.

'Francesca?' Krish's voice called out.

*Bugger.* When it came to people who she could call in a crisis, her list was short. Her parents lived in Spain. She had no close friends in London. That left her siblings. Neither of her brothers ever picked up on the rare occasions that she called them. Too busy leading their important lives. To be fair, she didn't pick up when they called her either. That left her sister, Donna—named after her godmother (another Olympian). Although Francesca and Donna weren't close, at least she had a car and only lived ninety minutes away.

That's who Francesca had meant to phone. Unfortunately, in her panic, her finger must have slipped and she hit Krish's number. He was listed in her contacts as 'DO NOT CALL EVER'. Right under Donna.

Her cheeks flushed and her stomach twisted inside her. She didn't want him to play at being her knight in shining armour. 'In here,' she called out.

He pushed open the door and his eyes snapped to her, darting up and down her body as though searching for signs of harm. He took a step in her direction. Francesca put down her bat and turned away. She randomly moved some papers on the desk, afraid that he might try to do something stupid like hug her. She attributed the jump in her heart rate to post-burglary adrenaline.

His voice edged with anger and concern, he asked, 'Did they hurt you?'

'I wasn't here.'

'What did they get?'

She filled him in.

He bent down and inspected the lighting stands. 'Insured?'

'Mostly.'

'What does that mean?' Standing up, he pinned her with his umber gaze.

'It means that most of the things I have are insured. I couldn't insure everything. Too expensive.' Unfortunately, that included her back ups. The urge to curl up on the floor and hide almost overwhelmed her. She fought it, forcing herself to stand straighter instead.

He shook his head and muttered something under his breath.

She crossed her arms. 'If you're going to be like that, then you can leave.'

Krish mirrored her body language. 'No way. We're packing up and taking your things over to my new office. Van's outside.'

'What new office?'

'I signed the lease yesterday.'

'Thanks, Krish. But I'm fine here. I told you I'm not working with you.'

He threw his hands up in the air. 'Francesca. The new unit is secure. It's alarmed. You can't leave your stuff here. Half your door is missing.'

Annoyingly, he was right. The thieves had done a great job of cutting through all her padlocks and they'd taken a chunk out of the door when they'd kicked it in. An emergency locksmith would be expensive. Money she didn't have on top of the cost of data retrieval and the pest control. *Damn.*

'Ugh.'

'Is that a yes?'

Neither of them moved, and after a pause, he said in a higher-pitched voice, 'Thank you, Krish, for dropping everything and coming to help me. I'm so grateful even though I'm really crap at showing it.'

She clicked her tongue and rolled her eyes, but the ghost of a smile hovered on her lips. He always knew how to make her laugh.

He continued in a deeper voice, 'That's okay, Francesca. My pleasure. What are friends for?'

'Thank. You.' She enunciated each word and performed a sarcastic curtsey. 'My saviour.'

'You're welcome,' he said, bowing over his praying hands.

She bet he was loving that he could help her. Another notch on his chivalric belt. This robbery wasn't leaving her many choices with the dent it would put in her savings. Even so, she said, 'I'm going to pay you rent money until I can get this cleared up.'

'Really, don't worry about it.'

'No, Krish, I insist.'

'If it makes you happy.' Blowing out a weighty breath, he dropped to his knees, crawled under her desk, and unplugged the remaining monitors. 'Let's get started. I've got boxes in the van.'

'Where did you get a van so quickly?'

'It's Connor's.'

'My goodness. The royal carriage! I'm flattered.'

By six o'clock they had finished packing everything into the sleek black van, out of place on a street full of jalopies and rust. Thankfully, everything fit. She hadn't accumulated much clutter, and even though her office was a mess, her equipment was well organised. The hardest part was carrying her things up and down the stairs before anybody broke into the van to steal what was left.

They made the short drive to Camden and pulled up in front of a white stucco building with black windows. Francesca got out to stand on the pavement. She crossed her arms as she examined her short-term workplace. If her old office had been designed by Eeyore —a depressing grey edifice—then this one was the work of Tigger: bright and perky, with friendly yellow walls visible through the front doors. She wouldn't admit it to Krish, but she could already feel some of the tension leaving her body. She looked forward to retiring her cricket bat, at least for the time being.

Krish closed the van door and stood next to her, hands in pockets. 'What do you think?'

'Well, obviously, it lacks the sheer majesty and professional vibe of my last office, but I suppose it will do. Temporarily, of course.'

'Of course.' His lip curled into a half-smile. 'Let me show you the space before we unpack.' He took out a key card and swiped it to open the door. 'I'll get one of these for you, too. Hey, Mick,' he said to the security guard sitting at the front desk, an older man with thick black glasses and spiky grey hair, reading a book.

'Hey, Krish,' he drawled. 'I picked up that book you recommended.' He held up a copy of *Cosmos* by Carl Sagan. 'Pretty trippy.'

'Good, isn't it?'

'This guy's like a prophet. How'd he know this shit?'

Leave it to Krish to be best friends with the security guard at a building where he just signed the lease yesterday.

'This is Francesca. She's going to be sharing my office space for a bit.'

A thrill ran up her spine. The reality of what was happening settled over her. She'd be seeing Krish every day, just like old times. Breathing the same air. Despite all her misgivings and the sour after-taste of the robbery, she quite liked the sound of that. It could be fun, just for a little while. The best part was that she was still self-employed and wouldn't owe him any explanation about her comings and goings.

'What's up?' she said to the guard.

They took the lift to the second floor, and Krish led her to a yellow door with a small porthole window.

He unlocked the door, pushing it open and standing aside so she could enter. Overhead lights flickered on, revealing shiny, polished oak floors in a spacious room. A few dark steel beams supported the sloped ceiling, giving it an industrial look. The radiators—radiators! Posh!—matched the beams in colour. On the far wall, there was a small fridge and kitchen area, complete with a microwave and coffee machine. Fancy. The soft, early evening light fell through four windows along the right-hand wall. Opposite were doors leading to two other rooms.

Krish had already marked out shapes on the floor with masking tape. 'So in this spot, I'm planning to create a lounge, you know, for meeting clients. I'll build a false wall to block off the view of the kitchen, but also it'll give me more space to display frames. Like a gallery. The viewing screen will go over there.' He pointed to the wall behind Francesca and then to one of the other rooms. 'The editing suite. You can set up your monitors in there. I'll get black-out blinds for the windows, so there's no light spillage...paint the walls mid-grey.' He jogged to the other room and held open the door. 'Storage in here for all the kit. I'll install extra locks, of course.'

'Of course.' He was bouncing around like a puppy. It made her wish that she could be part of this. It seemed so well thought out and grown-up. Very Krish. He obviously enjoyed shooting weddings, much more than she did. To her, shooting weddings was just the best way for her to make money right now and work around her body's limitations. She didn't really care about all that 'best day of their lives' stuff and 'capturing memories' crap. She did the job and she did it well, without getting emotionally invested. Maybe that made her a bit of a fraud. She frowned.

'What?' Krish asked, scratching the back of his neck like he needed her to approve.

'No, it's good. I like it. You've obviously thought everything through.'

'Well, not everything.' He paused and looked at her, eyes narrowing.

Francesca froze. Was this it? Was he going to ask her the question she'd been dreading? She tossed her hair and crossed her arms, waiting. 'What?'

Krish sighed and ran his hands through his hair to the the back of his head. 'Technically, I still haven't told Connor that I'm quitting.'

She kept her face blank so the relief didn't show. 'Why not? Chicken, McFly?'

He cracked a smile at her *Back to the Future* reference. 'It's complicated.'

'It always is.'

Folding his legs, he sat down where the couch shape was marked out on the floor. She copied him, sitting on top of a 'chair'.

'I've worked with him for five years. He trained me. I feel guilty leaving him.'

'Yeah, but nothing is forever. I'm sure he knows you'll go eventually.'

'I know, but they just got back from their trip...'

'Good time for a clean break then. A fresh start.' She picked at the edge of a piece of masking tape that was sticking up.

'He wants to try his hand at fashion while me and Stella run the weddings...'

She laughed. 'When did you become so good at making excuses, Krish? The guy I used to know didn't let anything stand in the way of what he wanted.' Their eyes met and the smile fell off her face. The moment the words were out of her mouth, she realised her mistake. Her thoughts rushed back to the night she'd left him. Back then, *she* had been what he wanted. Her words danced perilously close to the thing she didn't want to talk about. She would have to be more careful in the future.

Before he could say anything, she kept talking. 'If anybody can do this, it's you. And he's not going to disown you, Krish. It sounds like you two are close and...I'm sure he values your friendship. And if he doesn't, then he's not worth having in your life anyway.' Just like she wasn't worth having in his life. Just like she had taken his love all those years ago and thrown it in his face. No wonder he was nervous about Connor walking away. Francesca had already done him the disservice of proving that life didn't always go the way he wanted.

She tightened her hand into a fist, digging her nails into the base of her thumb. Guilt squirmed through her. She needed to get out of that room. If she was going to work in the same office as Krish, she'd have to try harder to keep things light.

With a yawn and a stretch to make her look more relaxed than she was, she announced, 'I've got to go.' There was a Bollywood film and a vodka tonic with her name on it. Tonight she'd watch something fast and furious, like *Dhoom*. Something with less romance and more fast motorcycles. Francesca was especially looking forward to the drinking part.

'Yeah, me, too. I've got to get the van back to Connor.' He stood up, his tall frame unfolding so that he towered over her. He held out his hand to pull her up.

Without thinking, she took it and immediately regretted it. Five years had passed, but she still recalled the feeling of those hands on her skin. Heat rushed to her cheeks as she had a sudden memory of making love under the *Bladerunner* poster on his bedroom wall. She wondered if he still had it.

As soon as she had her balance, she dropped him like a burning coal. Rubbing her hand on her jeans, she turned towards the door of the equipment room. She quickly packed up her camera bag and grabbed the cards with the data that needed recovering. The feeling that this was a mistake slithered back into her gut.

Being with him felt so natural, the equivalent of slipping into a cosy pair of pyjamas on a cold winter's day. Even on their first date, she'd felt at ease in his company; she could be herself in a way she couldn't with her family or other people. If she was a kite, then he was her string. To her, Krish meant stability, and she needed some of that right now—even if it came with a generous dollop of sexual attraction. At least she was five years older and wiser. She could handle it.

With her hand on the door, she glanced over her shoulder. 'Please thank Connor for the van. And also...thank you.' Her eyes dropped to the floor. Gratitude didn't come easily to her. She didn't like feeling like she needed help or owed anybody anything. She could muddle through on her own, thank you very much. As a strong, confident woman, there was no way that she would let her brokenness define her or make her weak. If there was one thing she'd learnt, it was that the only person she could truly rely on was herself.

But technically this specific situation had nothing to do with her health. The robbery was beyond her control.

'My pleasure.' He pretended to tip an imaginary hat towards her.

As she exited, she shot back, 'See you on Monday. And...good luck with Connor. You've got this.'

## 8

As KRISH CLIMBED the steps towards the Knights' front door, he gave himself a pep talk, reminding himself to be brief, direct, maintain eye contact, and not back down. He'd made his decision. Opening his own business was the next item on his plan. He had to stick to it.

Releasing one last deep breath, he rang the doorbell. Through the open window, he could hear the sound of Claudia's distinct cackle. *Shit.* He'd forgotten they were having a dinner party tonight.

The door swung open, revealing Stella in a loose, turquoise halter-top dress that showed off her skin, freckled from months of travelling in hot places. 'Krish! What are you doing here?' She smiled and threw her arms around him, planting a kiss on each of his cheeks.

He hugged her back with affection. He'd always liked Stella and thought she and Connor made a great couple. Seeing how happy they were had given him the final push he needed to get over Francesca and start looking for the right life partner. And then his sister had introduced him to her friend from yoga class...the rest was history.

'You look amazing,' he said. 'Glowing with health.'

'I know,' shouted Claudia from the hallway, 'isn't it nauseating?'

She appeared next to Stella in a chic black cocktail dress. 'You staying for dinner?'

'Um—'

'Oh, you must stay!' said Stella. 'There's plenty of food. And it's vegetarian! We have so much to catch up on.'

*More than you know*, thought Krish. 'Well, I guess I could...'

She grabbed Krish's hand and pulled him into the house.

In his pocket, his phone vibrated. He slipped it out and saw Jess's name on the screen. He'd left her a message letting her know that he was running late. 'Sorry, I've got to get this,' he said to his host, pulling his hand out of hers as he answered the phone.

'Hey, hun,' Jess said. 'Just checking on your ETA. How's your friend?'

'All sorted. But I had to borrow Connor's van and now I'm just dropping it off—'

She lowered her voice. 'Have you had The Chat with him yet?'

He glanced at Stella and Claudia, who were standing one foot away, watching him. Stella smiled.

'Um, not yet.'

'Maybe deep down you don't want to do this...'

Krish sighed. 'No, I definitely do. You need to trust me.' He was about to say he'd already signed the lease but then remembered Stella and Claudia, loitering awfully close. 'Listen they've asked me to stay to dinner. Will that cause you any issues?' He looked over at Claudia, who raised an eyebrow at him.

'That's fine. We weren't doing much anyway,' Jess said.

'Great. See you later.' He hung up and smiled. 'Sorry about that. Girlfriend.'

'Are you still with Jess?' asked Stella.

'Yup. Going on two years.'

Claudia gasped. 'Should we be buying hats? I haven't been to a good wedding in soooo long.'

Krish scratched at the back of his head and looked away.

She jumped up and down. 'Yes! That's a yes! When? Tell me all about it.' Threading her arm through his, she pulled him towards the dining room.

Claudia's husband, Magnus, sat lounging in a yellow velvet dining chair and pouring himself some red wine. Krish tipped his head towards him.

'Krish is getting married!' announced Claudia.

'Congratulations!' said Magnus and raised his Riedel stemware high.

Holding up his hands, Krish said, 'Well, I mean. Not yet. I haven't even proposed.'

Magnus pushed his floppy brown hair out of his face and leaned forward, his smile dropping. 'In that case, don't do it, mate. You're way too young.'

'Fuck off, sweetie. I'm the best thing that ever happened to you,' said Claudia as she refilled her own wine glass and sat down next to her husband.

Maintaining direct eye contact with Krish, Magnus shook his head almost imperceptibly and said, 'Of course, you are, sweetie. And that's a fiver for the jar.'

'Bloody hell.' She swigged her wine with mock despair.

Stella came in, carrying a bowl overflowing with salad. Krish rushed to take it off her and put it on the table.

'Oh, you don't have to do that,' she said.

He shrugged. 'Is Connor here?'

'Hopefully he's on his way.' She glanced at her watch and bit her lip.

When Krish had left him, Connor was about to head home. Why was he so late?

From somewhere else in the house, a phone rang and Stella dashed out of the room.

'So how are you going to do it? The proposal, I mean,' Claudia asked.

Without asking, she filled his glass with wine. He would much rather have a beer but didn't want to appear rude.

He took a small sip. Tonight he would need to keep his brain clear for his talk with Connor. 'Well, I've got tickets to Paris in three weeks. Jess has never been—'

'Connor's on his way! Just stuck in some traffic,' said Stella, carrying a platter of garlic bread into the room. 'He said to start without him, so I'm going to bring the aubergine parmagiana in.'

'Oh my god, I love your aubergine parm,' said Claudia, and then in an exaggerated Italian accent: 'Just like-a mama used to make.'

'Not my mama. She's not the best cook.'

'How is she by the way?' asked Krish.

'Pretending to be a surrogate grandparent to Dilwyn and Ula's baby boy because Connor and I won't move to Wales.' Dropping into a heavy Italian accent, she said, '*Stellina, you are denying me the God-given right of every grandmother to live near her grandchildren.*' She rolled her eyes. 'She forgets that she did the same thing to her parents. At least Dilwyn and Ula are getting free childcare out of it.'

Krish remembered Ula. She used to be Stella's cleaner before she met Stella's childhood friend, Dilwyn, and moved to Cardiff to be with him. Now she ran a highly successful YouTube channel reviewing sex toys and had a sponsored podcast where she interviewed older couples about their attitudes towards sex throughout the course of their relationship. It was actually really interesting.

'You're lucky,' said Claudia, 'I wish we lived four hours away from Magnus' family.'

'Can I help with anything?' asked Krish, feeling like a party crasher.

'Actually, yes, we need to set a place for you. Claudia, can you show him where the plates and silverware are?'

As Krish attempted to make himself useful, he checked his watch. He hoped Connor would be back soon, and in a good mood. This Conversation was going to happen, and it was going to happen tonight.

. . .

By the time Connor finally arrived, Stella had finished eating and was watching Krish demolish his second helping. She had always admired his healthy appetite.

'Hello! I'm home,' he called. Those words made her think of a 50s sitcom: the dad, coming in after a hard day at the office. The mother, dressed to the nines and making sure dinner was on the table. She looked down at her fancy frock and the full table and fidgeted in her seat. She did not want to be that woman.

'Sorry, I'm late.' He kissed Stella on the head and then sat at the table, reaching for the bottle of red wine.

'Back to the grindstone already, I see,' said Magnus. 'Coffers a little low after your grand tour?'

Claudia thumped his arm. 'Don't be vulgar, sweetie.'

Connor laughed, but Stella could tell he was just being polite. She slopped some food onto his plate. 'Did you get lots done?' she asked through a tense smile.

'Yeah.'

She cut her eyes towards him, expecting him to say more. When he didn't, she picked up her fork and then remembered that she'd already finished.

He dug into his meal with gusto. 'What happened with your friend?' Connor asked Krish between mouthfuls.

'We, um, moved her stuff into my...flat for now.'

Much as she loved Krish, Stella didn't really want to hear about his friend. 'So, how was the Valentina Vavilvek shoot today?'

Claudia almost choked on her wine. 'Every time I hear that name, it makes me think of vulvas.'

Undeterred, Stella drummed her fingers against the side of her leg. 'So...?'

Caught chewing, Connor waited until he'd swallowed and then said, 'It was fine.'

'Fine?' She could understand that he was tired, but he knew how she felt about Valentina. And all he could offer was *Fine*. 'That's it?'

She caught Magnus and Claudia exchanging a cautious look across the table, but she didn't care.

'What else do you want me to say?' said Connor, helping himself to some salad.

Shrugging with pretend nonchalance, she swirled her wine around in its spherical glass and said, 'I just want to know what happened.' She took a sip and skewered him with her eyes.

Connor huffed a laugh. 'Nothing happened. It was just a shoot. Right?' He nodded towards Krish for back up.

All eyes turned to Krish, who suddenly found an intriguing tomato stain on the table cloth. He scratched at it with his finger. Stella's suspicions bubbled.

She glanced at Claudia and jerked her eyes towards Connor. Receiving the message, Claudia nodded and leaned in. 'Yeah, Connor, why won't you tell us? Did she try to fuck you again? Ow!'

From the way Claudia jumped, it was obvious that Magnus had hit her under the table.

But the most interesting thing to Stella was that, when she turned back to Connor, he was actually blushing. She'd never seen him blush before, even when he'd dressed up as Dolly Parton to confess his love to her all those years ago. Connor Knight didn't embarrass easily.

'Oh my god. She did, didn't she?' Stella's wine glass thudded onto the table, spilling drops onto the linen cloth.

Sitting back in his chair, Connor assumed a relaxed pose. Stella wasn't buying it. 'No, of course not,' he said. 'Krish was with me the whole time. He's always with me on her shoots. Sometimes she just gets…over affectionate.'

Krish made a noise that vaguely sounded like agreement, but it could also have been the noise people make when they're being strangled.

Claudia elbowed Magnus. 'Is affectionate another word for adulterous?'

As though it helped his cause, Connor said, 'Actually, she and her husband have an open marriage.'

Stella barked, 'Yeah, because he's GAY.'

'We don't know that for sure.'

'Actually, we do. Tristan told me. He saw him at some exclusive gay bar in LA.' Tristan was her best friend and old dance partner from when she'd won the Open Latin Dance Championship, aged 18. He was also a sore subject in their house after he had a short relationship with Connor's brother, Michael, following their wedding. In a surprise turn of events, Michael had broken Tristan's heart for once, saying the famous model and Strictly Come Dancing champion just didn't 'have the same life goals' as him.

Magnus piped up, adding his own thoughts to the conversation. 'One of my Cambridge chums had an open marriage. They're divorced now.'

Angling her body towards Connor and gripping the stem of her wine glass with unnecessary force, Stella asked, 'So what happened? Did she hit on you?'

The question lingered as the whole room held its breath, waiting for Connor to reply. Only the sound of Grace's raspy snores crackled through the baby monitor, adding to the tension.

Finally, Connor sighed and said, 'Of course she hit on me. But I didn't do anything because I'm *happily* married. To *you*.'

The air in the room stilled after Connor's declaration, like the calm before a storm. Magnus was studying the contents of his wine glass; Claudia leaned forward onto the table as though waiting for Act Two; and Krish seemed to be playing musical statues, his whole body frozen while just his wide eyes darted from Connor to Stella and back. He wiped sweat off his face with a napkin. Stella narrowed her eyes. He looked guilty. Why did Krish look so guilty? What had happened?

She could feel a fight brewing inside her. She *knew* she was right about Valentina. The one time they'd run into her at a private members' club, the woman had pawed at Connor like Stella wasn't there. If she was comfortable acting like that with Connor's wife present, then what did Valentina do without Stella to hold her in check? She didn't care if half of Connor's income came from her: No more shoots with that...vulva.

Her mouth opened to say so, when another voice from across the table cut through the tense atmosphere: 'Connor, I'm leaving you to start my own business!'

It took Stella a moment to realise the words came from Krish. He had pushed his chair back abruptly and was standing, hand clamped over his stomach like he had food poisoning.

Claudia slapped Magnus on the arm. 'Ha! I was *not* expecting *that*.'

KRISH HAD HICCUPS.

His body sometimes reacted this way when he was under stress or disappointed with himself—and right now he was both. He sat in the kitchen staring at a porcelain chicken while Stella and Connor argued in the other room. Magnus was rocking a sleepy Grace in his arms after she'd woken up from all the shouting.

'Sex,' said Claudia as she poked her finger into the icing of the carrot cake they probably wouldn't get to eat. 'That's the best way to get rid of hiccups.'

'No—drinking water upside down while holding your breath,' said Magnus, bouncing gently while Grace snored.

'That's an old wives' tale. Never works,' said Claudia.

'Well, to be fair, sweetie, telling people to have sex to get rid of hiccups isn't the most practical of suggestions.'

'Worked for you that time in Mallorca.' She winked at him and clicked her tongue twice.

Krish wished he were anywhere but here. In hindsight, he could probably have chosen his moment better. But the words had burst out of him, a volcano choosing the worst moment to erupt.

He hiccuped again. He counted ten more ceramic chickens in

their kitchen before the next hiccup came. Why did they have so many chickens?

Stella barged into the room and prowled around the island as though trying to decide what to do. Finally, she headed for the open bottle of wine on the counter and drank straight from the neck.

'You okay?' asked Claudia, rubbing Stella's back.

A pointed, sidelong glance was the only answer Claudia got, as Stella took another long drink.

Krish hiccuped.

Putting down the bottle, she asked him, 'What swims in the sea?' The randomness of it surprised him.

He paused. What was the right answer? Was this a trick question? 'Fish?'

Stella looked at him and waited for a moment. 'Do you still have hiccups?'

The porcelain chicken seemed to be staring at him: *Well, do ya, punk?* Krish anticipated his next spasm, but it never came. 'That's crazy. How does that work?'

Stella shrugged. 'No idea, but it does. Connor wants to see you, by the way. He's downstairs in the gym.'

Suddenly Krish was very attached to his kitchen stool. He didn't want to leave it.

What had he been thinking when he blurted out his news during Vavilvek-gate? He had just wanted to help. It had temporarily done the trick, but then the argument had continued. And Krish had just felt worse as he realised poor Connor now had an angry wife and a defecting employee to contend with.

At least it was all out in the open now. Connor knew he was leaving and was presently in the gym, waiting to chat. After arguing with Stella. Perfect.

'Krish, you'll be fine,' said Stella, putting her hand over his. Ironic that she used the same word Connor had used to describe the shoot with Valentina. *Fine*. Krish agreed with her; it was a meaningless, nondescript word.

With a sigh, he climbed off the stool and trudged down the stairs as though going to the headmaster's office. He knew in his heart that everything would work out—it always did—but that didn't mean he was looking forward to the conversation.

Krish entered the small home gym—a room scattered with a few pieces of training equipment and some weights. Connor had changed into a sweat-wicking t-shirt and shorts. He wrapped his hands in tape before slipping them into a pair of boxing gloves.

'Hey, Boss.'

Without returning the greeting, Connor motioned towards the sparring pads with his chin, a wordless instruction to put them on. Bracing his feet for impact, Krish held up his padded hands and waited for the first punch.

The jab came hard and fast, followed by another and another. The pads absorbed the majority of the shock.

Punches kept connecting and Krish wondered how much longer this would go on before Connor actually spoke with him. His guilt over leaving grew with each hit, but so did his determination to go. Just because he felt guilty over something didn't mean it wasn't the right move. He had to do what was right for *his* future, for *his* dreams. Running his own business was the next step in his plan, followed closely by proposing to Jess. He only had one life to live, and there were things that he wanted: a successful career as a photographer and entrepreneur, a wife, kids…this conversation was the first step on that path.

With one final punch, Connor, now covered in sweat, dropped his fists, shook off the gloves, and picked up his water bottle. Krish slipped the pads off and tossed them on a bench. He took a deep breath and opened his mouth to speak.

'So, you're leaving me. When?' said Connor first, his voice gruff.

'I'm happy to work out my notice period.'

Connor took another swig from his bottle and wiped his hand across his lips. 'I'm not going to hold you back. If you want to go, then go.'

The edge of displeasure in Connor's voice punched Krish in the gut. He wasn't ready to be fully kicked out of Connor's circle of trust. 'I can still assist you at the weddings we have scheduled…and for shoots. I wouldn't leave you short-handed. And I'll keep replying to emails for you.'

Eyes on his water bottle, Connor toyed with the mouthpiece before letting out a huge sigh. 'I knew this day would come. You're too good…too talented, to stay with me forever.'

Relief that Connor didn't hate him whooshed through Krish's body and tears pricked behind his eyes. He had never been ashamed of showing emotion. His dad cried at romcoms and cat videos, so Krish had followed suit. 'Working with you has been one of the greatest honours of my life. You've taught me so much, and I wouldn't be half the shooter I am without you.'

'That's true.' The corner of Connor's mouth lifted in a cocky, half-joking smile. 'What are you going to do?'

This, Krish could talk about. 'Big, multi-day Indian weddings, offering a full service. Photography, video.'

'Have you written a business plan?'

'Of course I have. You taught me well, Obi-wan.'

They laughed.

Connor sobered and caught Krish's eye. 'Don't be a stranger, okay? If you need anything, you call me, anytime.'

Those tears pricked again. 'Yeah, Boss.' He stepped towards Connor with his arms thrown wide, but then realised that he was covered in sweat. Krish made 'air-hug' motions instead, mirrored by Connor.

He ran his palms over his face and sighed. 'This has been one helluva day.'

'Is Stella going to forgive you?' Krish asked.

Connor threw up his hands. 'She's told me I'm never allowed to do another shoot with Valentina again. But she'll come around when she accepts that one shoot with Valentina pays for one year of school for Grace. Private school fees are ridiculous around here. Almost eight grand per term.'

Krish had never heard Connor worrying about money before. Perhaps the six months away had put a bigger dent in their finances than he had thought. 'Is everything okay? Is the business okay?' he asked.

'Oh, yeah! Fine,' said Connor, wiping a towel across his face and throwing it towards the stairs. 'But if I'm going to take on fewer weddings while I build up my fashion portfolio, I need to make sure my family is provided for while I do it.'

That made sense. 'So no more shoots with Valentina, huh? Good luck breaking the news to her.' He didn't envy Connor that job. Valentina was spoiled and not used to hearing the word no. She would make it as difficult as she could for Connor to walk away from her.

Krish expected Connor to roll his eyes, maybe smile and make a joke. But he just took another sip from his water bottle and stared fixedly into the middle distance. Krish pursed his lips. He hoped Connor wouldn't do anything stupid.

A yawn unexpectedly came over Krish, and he hid it behind a fist. Today had been both emotional and tiring with the shoot, Francesca's robbery, and then this. He wanted to escape to Jess's flat for some TLC. 'So…we're good?'

'Of course we're good.' Connor clapped him on the back.

As Krish slipped out after saying his goodbyes, his desire to celebrate was tinged with a touch of worry. Would Connor and Stella be alright? Krish was walking away from more than just a job; the people who lived in that house were family. He was Grace's godparent along with Claudia, after all. The health of Grace's parents' relationship mattered to him.

He exhaled. He couldn't think about that right now. Instead, he pulled out his phone and texted Jess to chill the champagne.

## 9

MONDAY DAWNED HOT, but pain-free.

Every morning after she opened her eyes, Francesca would lie in bed for a few minutes and concentrate on each part of her body, determining where it sat on a scale of one to ten. Today, nothing. She blew out a sigh of relief, especially as the first item on her to do list was a session with her personal trainer—a perk paid for by her parents. She didn't like asking them for money, but when it came to her health and managing her symptoms, she didn't have a choice. So they paid for her PT, her nutritionist, and any other private health-care appointments that popped up.

Arms sore and clothes sweaty after her session, she trekked to Tottenham Court Road and a cramped, dark help desk at the back of a shop crowded with all things computerised. The technician, a hairy, heavyset man with supersized ears supporting the weight of his thick glasses, estimated it would cost £500 for him to get all her deleted wedding files off the cards—half of the price she had been expecting. Bonus.

Afterward, she hurried home to let in the pest control man, who set some traps and dropped poison under the cabinets. Job done. Take that, Ratty. Feeling like she'd already accomplished a lot, she changed into a pair of shorts and tank top and stuffed her computer in her pack. She decided to walk to her new office (42 minutes door-to-door). She liked to walk when she could, especially as she spent so much time at her desk, and besides, exercise was good for her symptom control. On the way, she mentally catalogued the rest of her To Do list, which included a backlog of weddings to edit and downloading a short registry wedding she'd filmed over the weekend.

At two o'clock, she picked up her new set of keys and a swipe card from Mick at the front desk, even managing some friendly small talk about the heat, then rode the lift up to her temporary office. As the lift doors opened, she heard the unmistakable, unpleasant cacophony of Peter Cetera's whiny singing voice inter-mixed with the whirr of a drill.

Before she went in, she peeked through the porthole window and had to catch her breath. Sawdust danced in the rays of sunshine coming through a skylight. Krish was building the partition wall he'd mentioned; bits of wood and boxes from Ikea littered the floor space.

And he was half naked.

Beads of sweat rolled down his skin. His back and shoulder muscles undulated as he sawed at a piece of wood and then hammered it to another. He swiped his forearm along his hairline before taking a long swig from a water bottle. Time had definitely dulled her memory of his torso. He'd always been muscular, but had he always been *this* muscular?

Somebody pass her a Diet Coke.

She took a step back from the door, mindful that she didn't want him to catch her leering at him. The suspicion that this whole venture was a bad idea barged into her thoughts, again. She chewed at her lip. Well, she was already here. No going back now.

Squaring her shoulders, Francesca stepped into the room and waited for him to notice her. 'Somebody's been eating their

Weetabix,' she quipped when his eyes rose up from his woodworking project.

'Hey, Francesca,' he said as he grabbed for a maroon t-shirt and slid it over his head. Ever the gentleman. She was tempted to tell him not to bother on her account.

'Sorry about all the mess.' He waved his hand to indicate the whole room.

'You still listen to this crap?' She waved her hand to indicate the cringeworthy music.

A smile rippled across his face, making her breath hitch in her throat. 'Chicago is the best band to come out of the sixties.'

'Au contraire, my friend. The Rolling Stones, The Doors, The Who…I know who I'd back in a street fight.'

He laughed and turned down his music. She pushed down the lingering tremor of attraction and made a beeline for the editing room. She wasn't looking forward to setting up her monitors and computer.

She stepped into the room to find it smelled of fresh paint, the walls already covered in the 18% grey colour perfect for editing spaces. Dark, Roman blinds blocked out the light of the only window. On top of that, a bank of white Ikea desks ran around the perimeter. Her workstation was already set up.

Francesca grinned. 'Krish! Oh my god. I could have done this. You didn't have to—'

'It's fine. I've been working flat out all weekend to get everything ready.'

'How did you get all this furniture here?'

'I rented a van.' He dabbed his brow with a small towel.

'Why didn't you just borrow Connor's?'

'Yeah…um. "Sorry, Connor, I know I've just left you in the shit by announcing that I'm quitting, but do you mind if I borrow your van so I can furnish my new office?"'

'Point made. But still, are you Dr Strange? Did you bend space and time to get this all done? Have you slept?' She just couldn't believe that he had done all this, for her. Lancelot to the rescue.

'Oh, Jess helped me. She painted the walls and built all the desks in there.'

Francesca bit the inside of her lip and nodded, her grin slipping. She quickly fixed it back on her face before he could notice. The other, faceless woman felt like a presence in the room. If Francesca had ultra-violet eyesight, she imagined she'd see Jess's fingerprints everywhere, even on Francesca's things. She wiped her hand across her keyboard, as though that would clean off any of Jess's DNA. 'Well...thanks.'

She carefully emptied the contents of her bag onto her new desk, plugging the extra monitors into her laptop and setting up the drive reader for her back-ups. Krish leaned on the doorway.

'Good weekend?' he asked and sipped from his bottle.

The wedding she had shot on Saturday had only lasted a few hours, a small affair, which was lucky for her because her uterus had not been in the mood. Each second felt like an hour when her endometriosis flared up, the unwelcome wedding guest. She'd already used co-codamol for four days that month, which was her self-imposed limit so she didn't get the unwanted side effects. She'd had to rely on ibuprofen, which generally wouldn't dull the discomfort of a paper cut, much less stabbing pain. It had been one of those days. She'd stayed in bed for the rest of the weekend. 'Good enough.'

He was silent for a second, as though searching for something to talk about. 'How's the family?'

Laughing, she said, 'Still crazy. Still over-achieving.' Her parents, ironically named Mary and Joseph, had met competing for Great Britain in rowing at the 1976 Olympics. Her father won silver while her mother placed eighth in the Women's Coxed Four—it was the first year women competed. Her dad's silver medal sat in pride of place in their house, along with all the medals earned by various Marches throughout the years. Except Francesca. She didn't have any medals.

'Are your parents still living in Spain? Seville, was it?'

'Yup.' The Holy Couple had emigrated to Spain the moment Francesca completed Sixth Form, as though their parenting tenure had come to an end, leaving Francesca to fend for herself. Her two brothers were in medical school at the time and her sister was halfway through law school. Francesca didn't go to university.

She didn't want to talk about her family. Even from miles away, they made her feel inadequate. 'How's your sister?' When they were dating, she'd gotten on well with his sister, Ankita.

'Pregnant, actually. Thirty weeks.' A big smile spread across his face and Francesca had to purse her lips to keep her chin from quivering.

He'd always wanted kids. He'd mentioned it within weeks of them starting to date. If anyone in the world was meant to have children, it was Krish. She'd watched him interacting with them in the wild: in parks, or restaurants, or even just walking down the street. He always squatted down to their level to chat with them, like they each deserved to be treated like intelligent mini-humans. Children gravitated towards him, as though they sensed his innate goodness. Kids were excellent judges of character. They never came near Francesca.

Ankita's baby would be lucky to call Krish uncle.

'Wow, give her my congratulations.' Moving her bag off her chair and sitting down, she said, 'Well, um, *lobster stew*, as they say.' *They* being a producer on a film she'd worked on briefly who had said it constantly on set. *'Come on, everybody! Lobster stew!'*, which meant *lots to do!* He insisted it was lingo he'd learnt on the set of a major Hollywood film. Yeah, lingo for *twat*. She wasn't sure why she'd repeated it. *I guess I'm a twat, too.*

'Well, let me know if you need anything. I'm just going to...keep building stuff.'

'I can help if you need me to...'

'Nah, I'm good.'

'Build it and they will come,' she quoted randomly, before putting her headphones on and diving back into the nauseating world of other people's happiness.

BY THURSDAY, KRISH HAD BUILT AND PAINTED THE PARTITION, AND real furniture now sat where the masking tape outlines had once lived. Some of his favourite shots of South Asian brides and grooms hung on the walls, the high gloss of the acrylic giving them a luxurious feel. Now he just needed some potential clients to dazzle into booking him.

His website was already up and running. He'd been working on it for months with a designer who specialised in sites for photographers. It looked pretty amazing, if he did say so himself. A black background with bright splashes of colour captured that luxury feeling he wanted. On the first page, there was a slideshow of hero shots of Asian couples. Bam! Visually, it said *Krish Kapadia is fucking awesome. Book him now.* The only problem was that *Kapadia Photo & Video* lacked half that capability: he didn't have a videographer on his books. Although he was in initial talks with a few people, nobody's CV leapt out at him.

And the one currently sharing his office was a no-go—even though he thought she was the most talented of the lot.

As usual, the thought of Francesca brought up conflicting emotions. He was happy to be helping her out, but felt guilty at the same time.

He'd already told two lies.

One, to his sister, whom he spoke with on his way to work that morning. If he had mentioned that Francesca (or as Ankita referred to her, The Succubus of Joy) was taking temporary sanctuary in his office, Ankita would probably be so angry that her baby would pop out. Despite the fact that Ankita and Francesca had gotten on well when he was dating her, his sister had lived through the aftermath of 'Fucking Norman' and would not welcome Francesca back with open arms.

The second lie he'd told had been over the weekend, while he and Jess readied the office. She'd asked about his friend, Francesca. He hadn't exactly *lied* about who she was; he just *omitted* some of the story. Francesca was simply an old friend in need, not the woman who'd broken his heart five years ago. Krish had never told Jess the whole saga of Francesca. When he'd met Jess, Francesca was three years in his past. Like curing hiccups, everybody had an opinion on what to do to get over heartbreak. Sleep around. Go out and party. Travel the world. Work out. For him, time and relegating her to his past had done the trick. When he met Jess, he'd closed a door and moved on.

Even so, his gut twisted whenever he thought about holding back from her. He was planning to propose in exactly three weeks. Hopefully by then, Francesca would have sorted out her office and cleared out anyway, making the whole thing a moot point. He had faith it would all work out in the end.

That being said, he was enjoying having somebody in the office with him, even if it was his super-fit ex.

They fell quickly into a comfortable routine. By the time Krish came in every morning, Francesca was already there. Once or twice he wondered if she had actually gone home, but her clothes had changed, so...yes? He knew that she was behind schedule with her edits, especially as her most up-to-date files had been on the stolen disks.

He'd also gotten into the habit of bringing her a coffee (black, not Starbucks) and a sugar-free snack. It was no problem to pick up something for her when he ordered his own. In return, she made him cups of tea and sometimes brought him an extra portion of the ridiculously healthy salads she made for lunch, usually involving chickpeas, quinoa, and kale. They were never enough to fill him up, but it was the thought that counted.

Today, they were each plugged into their separate editing stations, their backs to each other facing opposite walls. He had neglected his Photoshop work while he finished the office set-up and now had a lot to catch up on.

A pair of oscillating fans blew cool air towards each of them. The news kept reporting that it was the hottest July on record. Just his luck. Especially as it meant Francesca was dressing for the season: tank tops revealing her subtly muscled arms and body-hugging denim shorts that showed off her toned legs.

He remembered when they were together, she used to jump up into his arms and wrap those legs around him. Today, her dark hair was scraped up into one of those sexy, messy buns. During one of their tea breaks, she'd mentioned that she saw a personal trainer on Monday mornings and then performed strength exercises that he set her throughout the week. Krish had caught her doing squats while she waited for the kettle to boil. He didn't want to acknowledge the immediate, physical reaction he'd had to her thrusting up and down.

A tap on his shoulder made him jump. She stood behind him, holding out a mug, as though his imagination had somehow transformed into reality.

'Thanks,' he said, taking the mug from her and putting it on a coaster beside his keyboard. He slipped his headphones off and swivelled around in his chair to face her. 'How are your edits coming along?'

'Good. Just working on a Greek wedding I shot eight weeks ago. Have you ever shot a Greek wedding?'

He said he'd shot loads with Connor. Actually in Greece.

She sipped at her tea cautiously and flinched at the heat. She put the mug down. 'If I ever get married, I want a Money Dance. They were looping strings of £50 notes around her neck. Probably enough to pay for the whole day. Crazy.' Walking to one of the fans, she pulled on the knob to stop it oscillating and leaned over so the air blew into her face. 'What're you working on?'

Krish tried to ignore how sexy she looked with the wind gusting through wisps of her hair. He crossed his legs and picked up his mug. 'The Gangster Wedding.' She moaned in response. 'Have you heard from the data recovery guy yet?'

'No, I'm going to call him later for an update. Starting to get nervous. I'm supposed to deliver a five-minute teaser reel to the couple in four weeks' time.' She stood and turned her back to the fan. 'I don't want Chuckles to come after me with his shovel.' She laughed.

Krish could hear the nervousness in her voice. He shouldn't have brought it up. 'So tell me, when did you get into weddings? Are you still interested in making documentaries...?'

'Yes, of course, but unfortunately, I need money to eat. I tried working as a telesales operator for a while but...I hated working in an office...and it didn't really suit my skillset.'

'I can imagine.' The thought of Francesca cold-calling strangers all day amused him. The constant hang-ups, having to deliver the same spiel over and over, conversion targets. He laughed and raised the mug to his lips.

Francesca crossed her arms. 'What does that mean?'

'Nothing! You're just so fiercely independent, I can imagine that an office wouldn't be your favourite.' The last place he could see Francesca was a corporate environment, unless she was the boss. She lacked the patience and ability to bite her tongue that a good worker bee needed.

She unfolded her arms, pulled the oscillating switch on the fan, and returned to her chair. 'You're not wrong.'

Krish tipped his head to the side and regarded her. 'I think you're one of the most hard-working people I know. I'm not even sure you actually go home between when I leave in the evening and come back in the morning.'

'I do,' she said, her lips pushing to one side and her eyes to the other. A lie.

'I knew it!'

'It was only once! I just have so much editing to do. That couch is really hard, by the way.' She cricked her neck.

'I didn't buy it for sleeping on! It's not healthy to work 24 hours a day.' He sipped his tea. She'd made it perfectly: not too milky, no sugar. 'You know what you need? A hobby.'

She gave him an aggrieved look. 'I have a hobby. I have a personal trainer, remember?'

'That's not a hobby. That's more work. I mean something you do for fun.'

'I do plenty of things for fun.'

'Like...?' He thrummed his fingers on his desk like it would take her hours to come up with an answer.

'Like...none of your business. What do you do for fun?'

He raised his eyebrows and assumed an expression that suggested he was impressed with himself. 'Actually, I play the ukulele.'

That stopped her in her tracks. 'You're kidding me. Really?'

'I love it. I go for lessons and everything.'

'But you're so big and ukuleles are so...tiny.'

He smiled at the way she quirked her head to the side as though trying to picture him strumming away. 'Well, it seems to work. I'll bring one of my ukes in tomorrow and show you.'

'I'll be counting the seconds,' she said with her characteristic sarcasm before returning to her screen.


AN HOUR LATER, FRANCESCA WAS ABOUT TO ASK IF KRISH WANTED another cup of tea when his phone rang. She glanced at her watch, already knowing that it would be exactly 11:30: Jess o'clock. Every day, she stole five minutes to call Krish while her class ate lunch. Every. Single. Day. She would call again at 3:45. Francesca thought teachers were supposed to be overworked and time-poor. Apparently, not this one.

Jess's frightening efficiency was another thing that set them apart. Francesca existed in chaos. Krish didn't need that in his life.

She was about to go put the kettle on when Krish spoke. 'This is

Krish Kapadia,' he said, his tone business-like and efficient. Not the soft, low voice that he used on the phone to Jess. 'Yes.....mm-hmmm....oh, I'm sorry to hear that....are we available? It's short notice...just a moment. I need to check the diary.'

She watched as Krish sat back and revolved back and forth in his chair for a few seconds.

*What?* Francesca mouthed at him.

*Big job! Huge!* Krish mouthed back, followed by a wide smile. He wiped it off his face as quickly as it had come, as though the person on the other end of the line could see him. 'Yes, we're available on that date. Blenheim Palace, did you say?...Two-day event?...Yes, of course, I can do both photography and video. Not a problem.' He looked at Francesca and widened his eyes with intent. 'Yes, I'll reply to your email with directions to my office and we can meet in person to discuss...Sunday at 11:00? That's fine. See you then.'

He hung up and sat still for a moment, before exploding upwards to punch the air. 'Yessssss!'

'What is it? What's the job?'

Pushing his chair out of the way, he leaned over his computer and brought up an empty Google page. He typed something into the search bar and laughed when the screen filled with hits. 'I knew it!'

'What? Krish, tell me! The suspense is killing me.'

He moved aside so she could see his computer. The name he'd typed in the bar read 'Paramjeet Oberoi'.

She studied the image of a handsome Indian man, pictured with various women and/or fast cars. 'Oberoi...' she said. 'He's not related to Vashney Oberoi, is he?'

Vashney Oberoi was a huge Hindi film director, one of the biggest in Bollywood. The plot in the last Oberoi film she'd seen involved a cop whose Golden Retriever could sniff out criminals, but only if they had big boobs and perfect pouts. Romance and antics ensued, as well as a lot of dancing, including a number involving only dogs. Aside from being wildly impressed, Francesca had been wasted by the midpoint thanks to all the amazing over-acting, ridiculous scenarios, and big choreographed numbers. It epitomised everything she loved about Bollywood films.

For a moment, Krish's eyebrows dipped and he squinted at her. 'You know who Vashney Oberoi is?'

She realised her mistake and decided to go the blasé route. 'Doesn't everybody?'

He shook his head, moving on. 'Never mind. Just please please *please* tell me that you're available in four weekends' time.'

Her shoulder brushed his and her skin tingled. She shuffled away from him at the same time as he shot up to his full height. 'It's short notice,' she said, repeating what Krish had said on the phone. 'What happened?'

'Their original company can't do it. They double-booked themselves.'

'And they chose the other wedding over this one? Doesn't that make you nervous?'

He laughed. 'There is nothing I haven't seen at a wedding after shooting with Connor for five years. Can you please check your diary?'

She turned towards the wall where she had blue-tacked her kitten calendar and turned to August. The date was empty. But she was purposefully taking on less work as she eased towards the end of wedding season, so that she could finish all her editing by October before her operation. 'I'm available. But tell me about the job first,' she asked suspiciously.

'You *have* to do this job with me. Nobody good will have the date free at this late notice.'

Francesca crossed her arms. 'Gee, thanks.'

'Sorry, I didn't mean it like that. I mean…I don't trust anybody else to do as good a job as you. I already know your work.'

'Hmmm. Nice Recovery.' She glowed a little, knowing that he had such high regard for her skills.

'Do I need to beg?'

'Of course not. I'll think about it.'

'It's only in four weeks. The couple is coming here on Sunday to meet us. There's no time to think.'

His large, brown puppy dog eyes turned the full force of their power on her. She wanted to say no. She knew she should say no. It was on the tip of her tongue.

'Please, this is a huge break for me. If I play it right, I won't have to invest in marketing for years...*ever*.' He bounced up and down on his toes.

She put her hands on her hips and tipped her head back. She supposed she owed him a favour. He had taken her in when she needed it, and she didn't like having the debt hanging over her.

'Fine!' Throwing her hands up in the air, she smiled as she watched Krish's excitement. He took a step towards her as though about to gather her in his arms and lift her into a bear hug, but she stepped back. Recovering quickly, he danced around instead, pretending to screw in lightbulbs.

She sat in her chair, still smiling. She remembered this Krish: the joyful, goofy guy who'd won her heart all those years ago. Part of her felt glad that she could still give him joy; the other part was scared shitless. What had she just committed to?

Eventually Krish came off his high and sat down. He went to drink his tea, but spat it out when he realised it had gone cold. Putting the mug aside, he fished a notebook and pen out of a drawer. 'I know we haven't got the job yet, but you should start thinking about who you want on your team.'

'My *team*?' What was he talking about? She'd never run a team before.

'You'll need a second camera, maybe even a third...'

'Krish, how am I going to pay all these people? My bank account is almost wiped.'

'Francesca,' he swivelled towards her and leaned in, his elbows on his knees, 'after this wedding, you won't have money troubles for a *long* time. In fact, you'll probably be able to afford a new office altogether.'

She leaned back and crossed her arms behind her head. She liked the sound of that. Financial security was something she hadn't experienced in a while...if ever. And the idea of a new office was exciting, but...

'Great. I guess I'll be able to get out of your hair sooner than I thought.' She rotated her chair back to her bank of screens and willed the sudden wetness in her eyes to go away.

## 10

FRANCESCA PUSHED the door of her flat open and sniffed the air for the smell of decomposing rat.

Nothing.

She flicked on the lights and went straight to the cupboard under the sink to check the food compost bin. Inside, she saw the green biodegradable bin liner had been chewed all around the sides, evidence that the rat king still lived.

The bastard.

In the four days since the pest control company had been to drop the poison and set traps, the rat seemed to be taunting her, leaving mementos of his continuing freedom. A small black poo here, a pile of half-eaten crumbs there.

'*I'll get you, my pretty,*' she swore to the empty flat.

Dumping her bag on the floor, she flopped down on the sofa. Krish had pushed her out of the office bang on 5:30, telling her to go home and celebrate. She pointed out they didn't have anything to celebrate yet, but he assured her that he had a feeling everything would work out. Francesca laughed. She should probably believe him, the man who lived a charmed life, who no sooner thought that he wanted something than it fell into his lap.

So different from her life, just trying to survive from day to day. This week she had been lucky. Her pain had left on Sunday night and not yet returned. However, she was no fool. She'd learned from hard experience that it would be back, and soon. The longest she had ever gone without symptoms was nine days. Her current streak was four.

She had already looked at her calendar and counted out the days until the Blenheim job. She usually had a 28-day cycle, which meant she should be finishing her period just before the wedding. Fingers crossed that her body stuck to its own schedule for once.

Just in case, she'd save up her co-codamol days.

She had just started chopping a cucumber when the sound of pumping Hindi music started up downstairs.

*It must be fucking Thursday.* She skewered the innocent vegetable on her knife. Picking up her foot, she prepared to stomp on the floor.

And then stopped.

Krish's voice flitted through her thoughts: *You know what you need? A hobby.*

She lowered her foot as she considered the possibility. 'Nah,' she dismissed the idea and picked up the knife again. She couldn't do Bollywood dancing. What a ridiculous idea. Even so, her hips bounced to the music and her foot tapped.

The big choreographed scenes were the part she loved most in Bollywood films. Whether it was the swaggering, confident moves of Katrina Kaif or the sensual bellydancing of Nora Fatehi, Francesca appreciated the talent, passion, and sheer opulence of the dance numbers, which often took weeks to film.

She slid her phone out of her back pocket and found the website for the studio downstairs. The tagline read 'Walk-in classes for all abilities.' Well, that included her at zero ability. She clicked on the Thursday night class.

'Learn to dance like a Bhangra Babe with Bollywood choreographer Jaiveer Babu.' Curious, she tapped on his name. 'Jaiveer Babu is one of Bollywood's hottest young choreographers. His hook move from *Naach Utsav* inspired an avalanche of dance challenges on social media, and he received a Fanfare Award for his work on Vashney Oberoi's *Panje ka Nyaay*, where he choreographed a mind-blowing sequence featuring 100 dancing Golden Retrievers.'

'OMG!' Francesca couldn't believe it. She'd thought the studio below was just some poxy outfit that annoyed her with loud music every night, but there was actually some real talent teaching down there. And the fact that their teacher had worked with Vashney Oberoi felt like some sort of *sign*.

Should she do it? It would be completely unlike her and 100% out of her comfort zone. But maybe it would be beneficial to have something in her life besides work, health issues, and hankering after her ex-boyfriend.

She booked a place on the class before she could lose her nerve and changed into the most Bollywood workout clothes she had: gold leggings left over from a fancy dress party and a matching gold sports bra. Perhaps it looked more 1980s than Bollywood, but it would do the trick.

The class had started five minutes ago. Grabbing a water bottle, her phone, and her keys, she rushed downstairs, out onto the pavement, and into the lobby of the dance company.

At the back of the reception area, a large glass window revealed a room full of people stretching. Francesca cringed. Maybe this was a bad idea. The thought of being visible to people in the lobby scared her. She'd hadn't danced in a controlled setting since her parents allowed her to quit ballet, aged 12, after she threatened to hold her breath until they stopped making her go.

The receptionist looked up from her computer and said, 'Oh, it's you' and picked up the phone to call the manager.

'Actually, I'm here for the class,' said Francesca, pulling herself up to her full 5'2".

Not bothering to hide her surprise, the woman swept her gaze up and down Francesca's ensemble. 'Well, that's just made my day,' she quipped. With a dubious laugh, she checked Francesca into the class, directing her to go inside.

'Thank you,' Francesca said with a flat stare.

The room was warm; fans blew from the corners, their efficacy almost nonexistent. The atmosphere was thick with the smell of sweaty bodies masked by floral air freshener. Floor-to-ceiling mirrors covered two walls, the rest were plain white.

Francesca wished she weren't confronted with her own reflection almost everywhere she looked. She also wished she hadn't gone with the gold ensemble. She was the only one dressed like an 80s throwback. Everyone else wore regular workout gear in less metallic colours.

They were a surprising mix: lots of women of various races and sizes, two East Asian men, and a couple who looked like they may have walked into the wrong studio. The male, a heavily-bearded hipster with a bald head, was warming up in a corner by bending over to touch his toes. His girlfriend, who had her hand on his bum for balance, performed more balletic stretches.

A number of the young women seemed to know each other, gossiping as they reached their hands into the air and bent from side to side.

Somebody started clapping to get their attention. 'Everyone in their places for the warm up. Satya, you lead today.'

As everyone found a spot, Francesca spied the owner of the voice reflected in the mirror, gliding behind her towards the stereo system in the corner. This must be Jaiveer Babu. He wore black from head to toe. If Bollywood ever did a remake of *Grease*, he'd be a shoe-in for a T-Bird. His walk was arrogant and erect, yet graceful, like he could segue into a step, ball, change at any second. 'Come on, people! Places! We have a lot to get through today. I'm trying out some moves for a sequence in the next Hirani film, but don't tell anyone.' He winked at the room. It said, *Look at me, I work with famous people.* Francesca rolled her eyes.

As he plugged his phone into the music jack, she staked a place at the back of the room. She liked the anonymity of the back row.

Bhangra music rolled through the speakers and Satya, a doll-like twenty-something with a t-shirt that read 'Desi AF', led the room through a series of simple stretches. Francesca could handle these. Easy peasy. When the choreographer deemed that they'd done enough, he clapped his hands again and switched the track. The next song started: a regular beat backed up by the jingle of a tambourine and a male voice half-singing/half-intoning the lyrics.

The choreographer stood in front of the class. 'I'll just give you the first eight beats for now. Five, six, seven, eight—' He exploded into movement as a second voice joined the first in the song. His right arm shot out to the side with his right foot, then both his arms raised above his head. While his left hand stayed in the air, his right snaked down, ending near his bellybutton. He dropped all his limbs just as quickly as he'd started, like a puppet whose strings had been cut. 'Got it?' he asked.

*No!* Francesca hoped he'd demonstrate it again. Or another hundred times.

'Satya!' he commanded. She stepped into his place and counted the class into the movement, executing it perfectly. Meanwhile, Francesca just couldn't seem to get the beat right. It wasn't that she didn't have rhythm; she did. But they were moving awfully fast. The hipster next to her also seemed at a loss. The two East Asian guys had it down pat, as did all of the other single women.

The choreographer took his place in front again and demonstrated the next eight beats.

Francesca sighed. Perhaps it had been a mistake to come. This was going to be a long night.

Forty-five minutes into the class, and the teacher called for a break. Francesca had managed to do about 40% of the dance so far. When the people in front of her were facing left, she was facing right. When their arms shot up, her leg shot out. She ran for her water bottle and glugged it. Her hair was plastered to the side of her face, and she wished she had one of those 80s-style sweatbands to match her outfit.

'You. Goldie.' The choreographer's voice commanded from somewhere else in the room. Francesca saw him in the mirror and realised he was speaking to her.

She pointed at herself. 'Me?'

'Yes, you. I like your enthusiasm, but your dancing is very stiff.'

Unbelievable. She was already in trouble for incompetent dancing. Was he about to give her one of those tellings off, like Debbie Allen? *'You want* fame? *Well, fame costs, and right here is where you start paying.'* Francesca thought these classes were supposed to be for fun. It's not like she was auditioning for one of the female leads in *Devdas*, a Hindi film with an iconic scene where two women battled it out on the dance floor. Well, she wasn't going to take his shit. He was messing with the wrong lady.

She crossed her arms. 'What?'

He raised an amused eyebrow at her and said, 'Stop overthinking things. You need to just go with it, let the music move you.'

What did he mean by that? If she didn't think about it, then how would she remember what to do? 'It's not exactly like breathing, is it? I need to concentrate.'

'Try concentrating a little less. Feel a little more. Smooth it out.' His mouth settled into an expression that said, *'Do you always want to suck?'*

Her hackles rose. 'Okay, you're the expert. Show me.' She flopped her arms down by her sides, and gave him her signature impudent stare, pissing off teachers since Year One.

He chuckled and moved in front of her, so close she could smell the peppermint on his breath. 'Fine. I will.' Taking her wrists in his hand, he raised her arms above her head. 'Breathe in as you do the first move, then breathe out' —he brought her right hand down. 'Then in. And out.' He continued to demonstrate the breathing for everything they'd learned so far.

Francesca couldn't get a read on him. Was he flirting with her?

Were they having a Johnny and Baby moment? When he'd first entered the room, she would have pegged him as gay, but now she wasn't so sure. He kept catching her eyes and holding her gaze in a very come-hither manner. When he finished his demonstration, he winked at her and said, 'Think you can do that?'

'Pfff. I'll give it a go.'

In the second half of the class, her hit rate rose to about 50%, but she still wasn't going to be winning *Strictly* anytime soon. As the string of moves grew and grew, she felt her concentration waning with her energy. The last straw came at the end: they had to whip their heads around and she ended up with a mouthful of someone else's ponytail.

She was done. She couldn't handle any more dancing tonight.

The choreographer chose four of the best dancers to perform at the end so the others could record the sequence on their phones and learn the moves at home.

Francesca swore to herself that she'd practice this week and get the moves down perfectly. Next Thursday, she'd come in and show that smug choreographer what she could do. She'd claw her way to the top of the class if it killed her. Well, maybe not the top, but not the bottom, where she currently languished.

As she left the studio, Satya, the dance lead, called out that she hoped Francesca would come back next week. Francesca smiled. *Looks like you've just found yourself a hobby*, she thought.

## 11

STELLA PUSHED Grace's pram through the streets of North London as she made her way home from the zoo. This was her third time there that week, so she'd bought an annual pass. The attendant at the entrance knew her by name.

She couldn't wait to get back to work. Much as she loved taking pictures of Grace, Stella craved some time with her camera and a grown-up model, to create whatever took her fancy. If she didn't do it soon, she worried that the skills she'd fought so hard to hone over the last four years would vanish from her brain. The muscle memory she'd developed with her camera would fade. Already, she couldn't remember half the things she used to know how to do in Photoshop.

None of the nurseries where she'd waitlisted Grace had spaces yet. At last contact, Doodlebug Daycare had said there might be a place at the end of the summer. But no guarantees.

And because she had been away traveling for most of the beginning of Grace's life, Stella had no childcare network: no babysitters that she trusted, no NCT friends to rely upon, no local grandparents who could pop in to watch Grace for a few moments while Stella took a breath.

And Connor was already talking about having a second child.

The thought made her want to staple her legs closed, although that would preclude the one thing that was still going strong in their marriage. She sighed. Their communication wires seemed to be crossed lately, and it had all started with that stupid Valentina Vavilvek shoot.

She still shuddered when she thought about the night of the dinner party. After everyone left, she and Connor sat down to discuss what had happened. Apparently, Valentina had pulled him into another room under the guise of looking at places to hang a picture and locked the door behind her. After that, she'd thrown herself at him, but he'd pushed her away, explaining that he was married and he loved his wife very much. She still tried to convince him, but he was firm. Disappointed, she'd finally let him out of the room.

Stella reiterated that he must never do another shoot with that woman again. She didn't care how much money it brought in. He promised he wouldn't.

They'd sealed the promise in bed, doing what he did best, aside from photography.

As she lay beside him, watching his beloved chest rise and fall, she'd had another of her imaginary visions of doom, this time involving the Scandinavian mafia and a car chase. Did Scandinavia even have a mafia? She quickly looked it up on her phone. Yes, it was called the *Juggemaffian*. Great.

However, since their talk, Connor never seemed to be around, leaving early for his studio across town and coming back after Grace had gone to bed. After six months of travel, he was throwing himself into work with a vengeance. They didn't have money problems that she knew of, so she didn't understand what was fuelling it. She'd gone from having all of his time to having none of it, and because she wasn't involved with the business right now, she had no idea what he was doing. He could be shooting Valentina Vavilvek every day, for all she knew.

But she trusted him. Connor Knight may be many things—a little arrogant, a little selfish, and a little unaware—but he loved her. He wasn't like Nathan, the older, married man she'd had an affair with a lifetime ago. Nathan had been her charismatic boss and she had been young, ambitious, and too eager to please. He groomed her to have an illicit relationship with him by showering her with compliments, assigning her projects to keep her at work late, and then offering to drive her home so he could pour his heart out to her about his failing marriage and horrid wife.

Before the affair started, she remembered how he'd touch her leg when he dropped her off outside her flat, and the sly, inappropriate observations about her outfit choices when they worked side by side in the boardroom. It was no wonder that she'd eventually fallen into his bed, like the inexperienced idiot she'd been. And then when his wife found out, she attacked Stella in front of the entire industry at an awards dinner. Stella shivered. In hindsight and with the help of therapy, his *modus operandi* was easy to identify, but at the time she'd been like a moth drawn to a flame. Although she no longer felt guilty or responsible for it, she didn't like thinking about that period of her life.

A car honked nearby, snapping her out of the past.

Stella pushed Grace past a stylish cafe with tables on the pavement. A group of women sat outside, prams arranged around them, laughing as they breastfed their babies and drank their coffees and ate their pastries.

'Is anyone else getting little bumps on their nipples?' asked one of the mums.

*Yes!* Stella wanted to yell. *I have those!*

For a moment, she toyed with the idea of sitting down at the table next to them and falling into their conversation as they compared notes on their child's poo. But her natural shyness balked at the idea.

Instead, she continued on her way, wishing yet again that she had done NCT classes before having Grace. But both she and Connor had been working right up until the birth. They just didn't have the time.

She sighed again. As her mother would say: *'Il monde è fatto a scale: c'è chi scende, e c'è chi sale.'* —'The world is made of stairs: some go up and some go down.' Maybe Stella was just having a bit of a down moment.

Pausing to close her eyes, she let the hot sunshine give her some mood-enhancing Vitamin D. Suddenly she was transported back to the shores of Lake Kivu in Rwanda, where she had lounged on the beach with Connor and Grace not too long ago and talked about the future.

'Do you think you'll shoot weddings for the rest of your life?' she'd asked him.

His head rested in her lap and Grace sat nearby, playing with an older local child who seemed to have temporarily adopted her. 'I've been thinking about that a lot lately,' he'd said. 'I think I want to start shooting more fashion and advertising, fewer weddings. Less weekend work, so I can spend more time with you and Grace. I don't want to miss her growing up because I'm working too hard, like my dad did.' Stella refrained from pointing out the other reason his dad missed half his childhood—because he had too many girlfriends to entertain.

Instead, she stroked her fingers through his newly long hair and said, 'That would be great. Do you think you can do it?'

'Well, there's a lot of snobbery surrounding wedding photography. I'll have to find the right agent, someone who doesn't see coming from a wedding background as a problem.'

'If anyone can do it, Connor Knight can.'

He'd looked up at her then, shielding his eyes from the sun. 'And you?'

She'd been about to share that she was thinking of moving into women's portraiture, when the local girl laughed as Grace crawled away towards an abandoned ball.

Connor leapt up, and the moment passed. They hadn't spoken

about it since. In fact, all he could talk about was when she would come back to work to run the wedding business. Now that Krish was gone, that left only her.

Waking from her daydream, Stella found herself approaching the zebra crossing made famous by the cover of *Abbey Road*. As she followed in the phantom footsteps of John, Paul, Ringo, and George, she had to laugh. Would she be forever stuck walking in the footsteps of great men? Would she ever be able to crawl out of the long shadow cast by her amazingly talented husband?

She hoped so. She was a star by name, after all—*Stella* meaning 'star' in Italian—and she needed to shine. As Grace stirred in the pram, Stella promised herself to talk about her future with Connor soon.

## 12

KRISH SURVEYED the office for the millionth time. He wanted everything to be perfect for today's meeting.

Yesterday, he'd gone shopping with Jess. They'd bought a Nespresso machine and a fancy capsule presentation case, every type of tea imaginable, plants of varying sizes to bring life to the space, and designer pillows for the sofa. They'd stocked the fridge with soft drinks, beer, and individual bottles of Moët. Jo Malone diffusers gave the air a pleasant, citrusy tang.

The office exuded luxury. Professionalism.

He rearranged his sample albums on the table. Satisfied with their placement, he picked up the remote and hit play, just to double check that the slideshow of his work was ready to go on the new 75-inch TV. He watched Francesca's showreel as well. She really was good at what she did. She had a talent for capturing those moments between moments, where people were unguarded, where the real story lived. Her training as a documentarian shone through her work.

Krish reset the slideshow and showreel and glanced at his watch. Francesca should arrive in half an hour, and the clients in an hour.

All he could really do was wait.

. . .

'WE'RE *BAA-AAACK*!' PROCLAIMED FRANCESCA'S SYMPTOMS AS SOON AS she opened her eyes following a shocking night's sleep. True to form, her body had given her exactly seven days of respite before the cycle of hell started again.

At this point, it wasn't the pain that bothered her. That would start next week. This morning, she awoke with a foreboding, like she never wanted to get out of bed. Like she hated everyone. Like she could kick a puppy and not feel bad about it.

Pre-menstrual tension.

She pulled the covers over her head. Why did it have to happen today of all days? This was the week of her cycle where she generally tried to avoid other humans. And now she had to go into work and be *charming*. Might as well ask Cinderella's step-sisters to be *nice*.

*Come on, Francesca, pull it together.* She hoped she could avoid igniting this opportunity like it was doused in petrol.

*Yippee-kiyay, Mother Fucker*, replied her ovaries.

Her monthly schedule looked like this:

*Week one*: No pain! No PMS! She could pretend to be a normal, non-broken person. The time always passed too quickly.

*Week two*: Emotional PMS that made her question every relationship she'd ever had with anybody in her life, along with uncontrollable fits of rage at anything and everything, followed by uncontrollable crying. Words skipped her internal editor and exited her mouth with abandon and deadly precision. Seriously, Cersei Lannister would take notes.

*Week three*: Pain time, when she felt like her uterus was being stabbed by tiny, evil elves living under her skin with long knives.

*Week four*: Her period. She laughed when other women complained about cramps and heavy flows. Most of them didn't know *cramps*. They didn't know *heavy flows*. She could go through an entire box of pads in a day, sometimes wearing more than one. And tampons…there were days when she was bleeding so heavily that she had to use two supers at the same time. Once, her iron levels dipped so low from blood loss that she ended up in hospital. On top of all that, the pain from Week 3 leeched into Week 4, so she had to plan her use of medication carefully. She only liked to take co-codamol for a maximum of four days a month, and not necessarily on consecutive days. That way, she could avoid the worst of the side effects. She had learned that using too much co-codamol bunged her up, causing even more pain. Therefore, she had to gauge when she thought her agony was at its height and allow herself her strongest meds on only those days. Sometimes she got it right; sometimes she got it wrong. Ibuprofen did nothing for her. Vodka tonics on the worst days helped take the edge off.

Her parents never understood why Francesca hated sport. Being Olympians, they wanted their four children to excel in physical pursuits as well. Her oldest brother was an ultra-marathoner and a doctor. Brother number two swam for Britain in his late teens and twenties while he went to med school. Her sister, a divorce lawyer, spent her weekends running night-time relays with a team of other insane, super-fit people, and she had also run from Land's End to John o'Groats in ten days for charity.

Compared to them, Francesca was the quintessential black sheep, the family failure. She used to joke that her parents should have stopped at three. Her mother pointed out that they tried to, but the sperm and egg that became Francesca had other ideas, despite the fact that her father had already undergone a vasectomy and her mother was over 40 when she fell pregnant. Early expectations were that Francesca wanted to be born so badly that she must be destined for great things.

Ah, well.

Francesca used to enjoy running...until she turned fifteen and her periods started. When she told her mother about her pain, her mother said it was just a part of being a woman. Their GP said the same, his eyes turning cold and uninterested whenever she arrived for an appointment. 'You, again,' he said more than once.

She continued to harangue her parents, and finally, in her early twenties a year before she met Krish, they finally paid for her to see a private gynaecologist. That was when she got her diagnosis and found out she wasn't crazy: polycystic ovaries, fibroids, *and* endometriosis. The holy trifecta of uterine disorders.

'And you'll never be able to have children,' said the doctor brutally.

After her diagnosis, she started the long journey of trying to figure out how to manage her symptoms, and even more important, how to *live* with them—because they weren't going to go away. There was no cure.

Sometimes it made her so angry. Like today. Why did other women get to have normal bodies, while she got this broken one?

She took a deep breath and threw off the covers. She trudged into the kitchen to make a cup of coffee. A scratching noise under the cupboard drew her attention.

That fucking rat.

Rage bubbled inside her. If she caught that rat, she was going to tear it limb from limb. That rat was everything wrong in this world. That greedy little rodent had already cost her so much money. So far, the poison trays went untouched, the traps empty. Well, she would take care of it herself.

With the speed of a Power Ranger, she whipped open the cupboard, surprising the furry beast. It was eating a crust of old toast on top of the food waste bin.

*Die, King Rat.*

The little white diamond on its forehead twitched in the moment it took for her to lunge at him. The food bin went flying, its contents spilling out onto the floor. The rat jumped back and disappeared down a secret passage. The pest control man said he'd filled all the holes, the liar.

Francesca swore, her breaths coming in fast huffs, the detritus of yesterday's curry and rice dinner staining her bare feet yellow.

Then the tears came. She wiped them roughly with her sleeve.

What the fuck was she doing? She couldn't be the person Krish needed her to be today. She would fail him. She would fail herself. She wasn't a good enough videographer to shoot this wedding with him. She would ruin their tenuous friendship, and he would hate her.

But she had to go. Francesca had sworn long ago never to let her own limitations get in the way of her commitments. Besides, she needed the money. Squeezing the edge of the countertop, she breathed in for ten and exhaled for ten.

She would get dressed. Put on some make-up. Brush her hair. And fake a smile like her life depended on it.

KRISH LOOKED AT HIS WATCH AGAIN. THE CLIENTS WOULD BE COMING in fifteen minutes, and Francesca hadn't arrived yet. He sent her another text.

**Hey, getting worried. Let me know your ETA. K**

He decided not to sign off with an X.

Wilting despite the fans, he rolled up the sleeves of his white Oxford shirt and smoothed his hands down his grey suit trousers. Casual, but professional.

If they booked this wedding, it could be the making of his business. Indian families talked. The bride and groom would have friends and cousins getting married, and they would need someone to capture it for them. He made a mental note to pack his new business cards in this camera bag for when people asked for his details at the wedding.

Examining the room one last time, he rubbed his hands together. It looked good. He'd set up an armchair on either side of the sofa: one for him and one for Francesca. The couple would sit in the middle.

The lift pinged. He hoped it was Francesca rather than early clients. The door pushed open and Francesca fell through, large sunglasses covering her eyes. She wore a black blouse and black culottes, a stylish combination. He smiled, happy that she had made such an effort.

'Sorry I'm late,' she grumbled. His smile faltered. Was she hungover? He had taken precautions to make sure he was well-rested for today, even sleeping alone at his own flat instead of hanging out with Jess as he normally would on a Saturday night.

'Are you okay?' he asked, his eyebrows pulled down in concern.

'I'm fine,' she snapped at him.

*Okaaaaay.* Obviously somebody had woken up on the wrong side of the bed.

'Would you like a coffee?' Perhaps some caffeine would help brighten her up.

'I can make it myself.'

She disappeared into the editing suite and emerged moments later without her bag or sunglasses. She had done her make-up, her eyes outlined in black and her lashes spiked with mascara. Between that and the shimmer on her lids, the effect made her eyes pop, the green pupils standing out. He could see that she'd applied concealer, too, but it didn't fully cover up the dark circles beneath.

'What?' she barked at him.

'Nothing. Nothing. I was just thinking that your eyes looked nice.'

'I don't need your approval.'

Whoa. What had happened to Francesca? She could be sarcastic and blunt, but this person was plain stroppy. Would she be able to get it together before the clients arrived? He was starting to worry about the upcoming meeting when the lift pinged again. His head whipped towards the door. 'They're here.' Too late for second thoughts.

He prayed, stuck a smile on his face, and went to greet them.

IT DID NOT START WELL. AND THEN IT GOT WORSE.

Francesca watched as the infamous Paramjeet Oberoi and his

fiancé, Ishani, glided into the office. Everything about him screamed 'spoiled wanker'. He was chewing gum with a vengeance, mouth open, one of Francesca's particular pet peeves. *Snap, snap, snap.* He wore a loose black jacket and skinny black jeans with a tight white t-shirt. A thin gold chain looped around his neck. His meticulously sculpted hair rose two inches into the air before tipping to the right, like a wave permanently on the cusp of breaking. His eyes were hidden behind a pair of Tom Ford sunglasses.

Francesca disliked him on sight.

She had done some research on him. Like her, he was the youngest of four over-achieving siblings. His eldest brother was the heir apparent, also a big-time director and the son being groomed to take over the family business. His sister was a huge Bollywood actress who had recently crossed over into Hollywood films. The third sibling, also a brother, designed all the clothes for the studio's productions and had a couture line of his own. And Paramjeet...he hadn't quite found his purpose in life yet. All the online pictures of him were taken at parties with a different girl on each arm, or at automotive shows modelling with supercars.

Paramjeet and Francesca may have both been the youngest members of their families, but whereas Francesca worked hard for everything she had, Paramjeet was a Bollywood nepo-baby who had opportunities handed to him on a plate.

She had looked into the bride, too. Ishani worked in entertainment law, like Krish's sister. Frankly, Francesca failed to see why somebody successful and motivated like Ishani would want to marry someone spoiled and dull like Paramjeet, unless it was the money.

Her opinion of him didn't improve when he studied his chunky watch just enough time to make sure everyone identified it as a Rolex and demanded, 'Is this going to take long? We've got somewhere important to be.'

Krish smiled like Paramjeet wasn't a dickhead and said, 'No more than an hour.' He held out his hand. 'I'm Krish—'

Paramjeet sailed past and left Krish's hand hanging in the air, which made Francesca's blood boil. The wanker plopped himself down on the sofa like an emperor, arm possessively thrown across the back. Krish caught her eye and let his amusement show just for a second, to let her know he wasn't bothered before smoothing his features over again. Francesca had to give Krish credit for his self-control and positive outlook. Personally, she wanted to smack the guy.

Ishani stepped into the breach, taking Krish's hand in hers. 'I'm Ishani. Sorry—I should have said when we spoke that we only have half an hour. There's a helicopter waiting to take us up to Silverstone.'

The bride was stunningly beautiful, with the kind of shiny, gravity-defying hair that would make a Kardashian weep with envy: midnight black and styled into a sleek over-the-shoulder cascade. Her nails were polished to perfection: deep, glossy red. Over her all-cream outfit, an expensive jacket perched on her shoulders like it wasn't sweltering outside. Francesca twitched. People who wore all white when it wasn't a wedding set her teeth on edge.

'No problem,' Krish said, 'we can be quick.' He gestured for Ishani to take a seat. She settled herself onto the sofa, placing a large handbag between her and Param-jerk with a braided gold handle that could probably pay off the debt of a small country.

Krish sat in his chair. 'Can we get you something to drink?'

'Coffee. Black,' said Param-jerk while Ishani asked for bottled water.

'I'll get it!' Francesca needed some space before she said something she'd regret.

Behind the partition where they couldn't see her, she took a moment to collect herself, shaking her hands out and rolling her head in a circle. She heard Krish make small talk about Silverstone, Formula One, McLaren, Lewis Hamilton. Nothing like fast cars for bringing men together. The groom actually laughed and his tone became less aggressive. She had to admire Krish's ability to get people on side.

Approaching the kitchenette, Francesca frowned at the new Nespresso machine in consternation. How the fuck did this work?

On the other side of the partition, Krish started the sales spiel. He'd talked her through it the other day, as taught to him by Connor Knight.

First, find out about the couple and what they wanted.

'I just want somebody who's going to make me look good in every picture,' the bride said. Francesca couldn't help but roll her eyes. She imagined that Ishani would photograph well in a dingy call centre with fluorescent overhead lighting.

Paramjeet finally piped up. 'We want photos and videos that look like one of my father's films. Better, even. And how can you fail, with two people as beautiful as us?'

'*Jeet!*' scolded the bride.

'Well, it's true.'

Francesca pretended to gag as she opened the luxury box of coffee capsules. She was confronted with five colour-coded rows: blue, red, yellow, black, and green. Being a fan of the *Matrix*, she decided to choose between blue and red. She thought Param-jerk was more of a blue pill kind of guy; he would choose wilful ignorance. She plucked the capsule out of the box and confronted the machine. Now what?

She lifted up a silver lever as she heard Krish move onto part two: selling what Francesca and he could do for the couple. He suggested they peruse his sample albums and she heard the soppy, dramatic background music from his slideshow start up. She slid the capsule into the hole and pressed a blinking button. Nothing happened.

'Oh, that's amazing,' she heard the bride croon. Krish *was* an amazing photographer. These rich wankers would be lucky to have him. Francesca stabbed at the button a few more times, until a groaning noise emitted from the machine. Something was happening.

Ishani asked, 'Have you shot a wedding at Blenheim before?'

Francesca huffed. Did it matter? A venue was a venue.

The groaning noise stopped and there was a moment of silence before black liquid spewed forth. 'Shit!' yelled Francesca as coffee splattered all over the table and dribbled to the floor. She'd forgotten to put an actual mug below the nozzle. She grabbed the first thing she could find to catch the liquid: a Jo Malone diffuser. She pulled the sticks out and tried to line up the small hole at the mouth of the bottle with the stream of coffee. A few drops burned her hand, but thankfully, most of it had already ended up on the floor and the stream sputtered out. She winced at the layer of dark liquid now sitting on top of the expensive oil in the bottle.

'All okay?' Krish called to her.

'Fine!' she barked back.

*Let's try that again*, she thought. She procured another blue capsule, inserted it into the machine, and opened the cupboard above to find a mug. She could see that Krish had stocked it with designer porcelain, printed with stunning Fornasetti faces. And she would really have loved to serve Param-jerk his coffee in one of those, but her hand strayed to the left, to a mug she had brought from home. It featured a still of a topless Ryan Gosling in the film *Crazy, Stupid, Love* next to Emma Stone's quote: 'Fuck! Seriously! It's like you're Photoshopped?!'

Francesca smiled for the first time that day.

Once it had filled with coffee, she organised the mug, a bottle of Evian, a glass, and a plate with some fancy biscuits onto a tray, and brought them into the viewing area. Krish moved one of the albums out of the way, and she placed the tray on the table. She watched as Param-jerk picked up the mug. He paused for a second as he read the quote and looked at the picture. Then he smirked at Francesca. 'Yeah. I get that a lot.'

His mask of amiability slipping, Krish's mouth hung open as he took in what she had done. She sat down in her chair and ignored him.

Recovering himself, Krish started the showreel of her work. She wished she could close her ears. She hated being reminded of all those weddings she'd shot. The one playing right now had taken place in central London at a snooty hotel. She remembered being in excruciating pain and having to run out to vomit in between speeches.

Sitting back in her chair, she rested her elbow on the arm and placed her middle finger across her lips, her pointer finger laying along the side of her face. Anyone looking at her would see a woman in a thinking pose, but really she was trying to cover up the tension building in her jaw. She ground her teeth together.

Ishani directed a question towards her. 'Have you shot any Indian weddings before?' Francesca's showreel didn't include any because the answer was no.

Francesca didn't trust herself to speak right now, so she just kept her mouth clamped closed and shook her head.

'Ummmm,' Krish said, jumping into the uncomfortable silence, 'Francesca *hasn't* shot any Indian weddings yet. We've only just started working together, but I can assure you her work is top notch.'

'I want drone footage and lots of tracking shots,' Param-jerk said with the vague filmic knowledge of someone whose dad worked in the movies.

*Shit*, she'd have to find a drone operator for her team. Did she know anybody? 'No problem,' she managed to strangle out.

'How many guests are you having?' asked Krish, in what she realised was an effort to draw their attention away from her. Thank bloody fuck for that. But instead of relaxing, her body stiffened with tension. She hoped this meeting would end soon.

'Five hundred for the ceremony and then another five hundred in the evening,' said Ishani.

That would make this the biggest wedding Francesca had ever worked. She must have made a noise because the bride turned towards her. 'I know, right? It's not that big, but we'll have the real wedding back in India in October.'

Gum snapping, Param-jerk added, 'Yeah. If you do a good job on this one, then we can talk about the next one.'

*Not for me,* thought Francesca. *I'm busy in October.*

A movement caught her eye. A small beige head poked out of Ishani's bag, and Francesca jumped. 'Sweet Christ!' she exclaimed. It whined, as though upset at the profanity.

Ishani lifted a small orange Pomeranian out of her bag and addressed it in a childish voice. 'Oh my little Fufu! Are you feewing left out?' She held up the dog and rubbed her nose against its wet nose.

Param-jerk, softening into a different person, took the fluff ball and cradled it like a baby. 'There's my girl!' A little pink tongue whipped out and licked him on the lips.

He settled Fufu onto his lap. Placing her hand on top of the rodent-sized animal, Ishani said, 'Fufu's our practice baby.' She laughed like it was funny. 'We'll definitely want some photos with her at the wedding.'

*Practice baby?* Francesca fought the urge to roll her eyes and lost. Practice baby. *Fuck off.*

She turned her head to study the couple. They looked like two people who had everything in life handed to them, who never had to deal with real problems. Their clothes, their mannerisms, their accents, their perfect dog. Francesca had worked with people who lived on the streets, who had been sexually assaulted at work, who had lost their jobs and not known where their next meal would come from. These two snobs would crumple under the pressures of the real world.

Francesca could feel her rage growing quietly hotter. Her breathing became more shallow as she struggled with her inner beast.

Sometimes she keenly understood the inequality of life. Did this couple ever stop to consider how lucky they were simply to have found love? They didn't have to consider chronic pain and their fertility before saying 'I do'. They got to have a 'Practice Baby', with the expectation of a real one down the line. Why did she have to wait for her life to start while this prick and his fiancée had everything fall into their entitled laps?

*Divorcees*. That was Francesca's plan. Right now, she would wait. While her contemporaries coupled up, married, and started families, she would wait. Wait for the separations and divorces. Wait for the men who already had all the kids they wanted, who were looking for an acceptable step-mother for their darling children. Maybe she could be that step-mother. With her tender nature and strong maternal instincts, she'd be a perfect fit.

She huffed with sardonic mirth and sliced her gaze away from the couple. Who was she kidding? Those kids would probably call her step-monster behind her back and make voodoo dolls with her face at summer camp.

But slotting into a ready-made family might be the only way she could get one of her own, the life she desired—the life that these two trust-fund babies so effortlessly took for granted.

She envied them their carefree love and their 'Practice Baby'.

The words came out of her mouth before she even realised that her lips had opened. 'You don't deserve to be this fucking lucky.'

## 13

KRISH BLINKED. What the bloody heck did she just say?

The room went silent and even the dog seemed to freeze. To her credit, Francesca also looked horrified at what had just come out of her mouth: her eyes stretched wide and she pursed her lips as though trying to imprison further words inside.

'Well,' said the bride.

'What did she say?' asked the groom.

Frantically, Francesca locked her gaze on Krish. He got the impression she was willing him to smooth things over, but there were limits to his charm.

'Um.' His mind went empty as a white board, waiting for ideas. What magic words would make 'You don't deserve to be this fucking lucky' sound like a sane thing to say?

His eyes fell on the Pomeranian, who raised an eyebrow at him and panted. Even the pooch wanted to know how Krish would get out of this.

Then it came to him. The only thing he could think of that might make this canine-loving couple sympathetic towards her. He rearranged his face into the picture of concern. 'Her dog died yesterday!'

Ishani gasped and Paramjeet hugged Fufu closer. They all turned towards Francesca, including Krish, whose eyes begged her to play along.

A moment's pause. Krish held his breath, unsure if she'd run with his ruse. He hated lying, but he had no other ideas to reverse her epic blunder. His mental white board said DOG in big, black marker.

Her bottom lip quivered, and she started sobbing. Her shoulders shook with grief. Salty tears wandered down her cheeks. She even managed a shuddering breath *and* a plaintive sigh. He'd never realised that Francesca was such a good actress; she was *nailing* this role. Ishani's eyes melted with sympathy and even Paramjeet was nodding his head, full of understanding. Krish struggled not to break into a relieved smile.

Francesca took a tissue from a box nearby and honked into it. 'I'm so s-sorry,' she said. Without another word, she shot to her feet and ran into the editing room, closing the door behind her.

'Poor woman,' said Ishani, turning her head towards Krish. 'What kind of dog was it?'

What kind of dog would Francesca have? The only one he could think of in that moment was—

'A doberman. Cujo. Such a sweet, *sweet* dog.' Was that the best he could do? Give Francesca an imaginary pet named after a murderous character in a Stephen King novel? His mental white board was shit.

They were both taking turns to hug Fufu like she might drop dead at any second. Now Krish really needed to bring the conversation away from dead dogs and back to weddings. 'Listen, I know Francesca may seem a little emotional today, but it's that same emotion that makes her passionate about capturing weddings with care and...such, such *feeling*.' Wow, the bullshit was flowing thick and fast now, but they were both nodding along, so it seemed to be working. 'We would love to shoot your wedding, so how about it? Shall we sign the contract?'

. . .

KRISH WAVED GOODBYE TO PARAMJEET AND ISHANI.

He *thought* he'd smoothed things over, but when he'd tried to close the deal, they insisted they still had to speak with one more company, for comparison's sake. He worried that it was a brush off. When they left, the bride was smiling, so that was a good sign. She promised to let him know by the end of the week.

After the lift doors closed behind them, Krish leaned his hand onto the wall and let his head sag. *What the hell had that been about?*

He hiccuped. Great, just what he needed.

Francesca was still hiding in the editing room. Krish stared at the door. He had no idea what he'd find in there—a raging beast? Broken computer screens? Francesca, stuck to the ceiling, like in *The Exorcist*?

She'd probably just caused him to lose his first lead. Since she fell back into his life, he'd done nothing but try to help her. Why had she done this? And what had been up with that mug? His anger flared, followed by another hiccup.

Running his hands through his hair and pushing up his sleeves, he took a deep breath before throwing open the door, ready to have it out with her.

And was met with tears. The shock of it was enough to make his hiccups disappear.

Francesca sat at her desk, trying to stifle the noise of her sobs by shoving a fist up against her mouth. The effort had turned her face red. Her shoulders shook. Black streaks crawled down her cheeks.

He thought she'd been acting when she started crying in front of the client, but it had been real. His anger melted away, replaced by guilt, his heart clenching as he thought about her crying alone in here for the last fifteen minutes.

Without hesitating, he covered the distance between them in two strong steps and pulled her into his arms. 'Chezzy,' he said, using his old nickname for her. He had never seen her cry like this. Not even when they'd watched *Beaches* together. Not even the night they'd broken up. *Fucking Norman.*

She buried her head into his chest and bunched his white shirt in her fists. He rubbed his hand over her back and made shushing noises. Francesca was in full sob mode. 'I'm s-so so-ho-ho-rry,' she croaked, her voice rough with tears.

'It's okay. I think I got things back on track.'

'Of c-c-course you did.'

He thought he heard a hint of a smile in her tone. He pulled back to look at her face and noticed the black streaks had transferred to his shirt.

Francesca saw it, too. 'Sorry!' she wailed and then starting sobbing again. She dug her head back into his chest, and he stroked her hair, remembering the way he used to curl it around his finger when they were in bed and then let it go, watching it become instantly straight again. He never did that with Jess, despite her long blonde hair. He wondered why. Probably because she already had curls.

They stood like that for a few minutes, letting her get it all out while he rocked her gently in his arms. Eventually, she stopped trembling and got her crying under control. He went to pull back to look at her face again, but she tugged at his shirt and said, 'No! I have to tell you something, and I won't be able to do it if you're looking at me.'

That sounded ominous. He let his hand continue to stroke her back. It felt so natural. 'Okay, I'm listening,' he said.

'About today. I know you probably won't believe me, but it wasn't my fault. I get really bad PMS. I mean, *really really* bad.'

Krish had grown up with a mother and sister. He didn't remember his even-keeled mother ever having fluctuating moods, but Ankita did get tetchy once a month. Correction: she got *more* tetchy than normal. But what he witnessed today? It was a whole new level.

Sifting through his memories of five years ago, he tried to recall if he'd ever seen her act like this, but came up with nothing. 'When we were together…?'

'I just *didn't see you* when I had PMS. I h-hid it from you.'

He supposed that wouldn't be too hard to do. He had vague memories of her cancelling a few dates due to work commitments. 'I don't mean to pry, but have you seen a doctor?'

She snorted and then sniffed. 'Several.'

'And there's nothing they can do?'

'Tried anti-depressants but they didn't agree with me. Made my insomnia worse. Now I just try to eat healthy, do my exercise, and ride it out.'

'Hmm. How's that working for you?'

She barked a laugh.

Tucking some hair behind her ear, he said, 'Well, there has to be something we can do to fix it. You can't live like this.'

She sniffled again. 'This is my life, Krish. And I can't be fixed.'

The sadness in her voice broke his heart. Krish was at a loss for words. What a horrible thing to have to deal with, like having a traitor inside controlling her moods. All he could do was hug her tighter. She had relaxed her grip on his shirt, and now her hands rested on his hips. He continued to run his hand over her hair, his thumb stroking her temple. Their bodies swayed gently together, like they were doing a slow dance.

Her crying had completely stopped and her breathing grew calm, even. He could smell the familiar shea butter and berries perfume from her shampoo, reminding him of happier times between them. Subtly, the mood in the room shifted from comfort to something else. Heat spread between them. Her hands tightened on his hips. On the topic of traitors living inside bodies, his own grew hard. He knew she'd be able to feel it through their clothes, and he closed his eyes. There was nothing he could do about it.

He remembered a walk they'd taken in the forest during a camping weekend. To kill the time, they'd been listing the top ten sex scenes in films, and the mood to create their own came upon them both. They'd found a quiet area enclosed by trees, and she'd jumped up into his arms, and they made love against the bark of a pine tree, the smell of evergreen and the noise of birdsong around them. When she came, he'd covered her mouth with his own, in case anyone was walking nearby. The whole scene had been worthy of a Hollywood film. Thinking about it now did nothing to help his current situation.

He should break contact. Walk away. But he was enjoying the sensation of her in his arms. A greedy part of him wanted to keep holding her, wanted to kiss her, or at least fantasise about kissing her. Fantasising couldn't hurt, could it? Just for a few moments longer. Then he'd step back.

The sound of the office door clicking open cut through his thoughts. 'Hello?' asked a female voice.

It took him a moment to realise it was Jess.


ONE SECOND THEY WERE HUGGING, AND FRANCESCA WAS STRUGGLING not to react to Krish's obvious desire pressing into her. It made her forget all about her PMS and gave her all kinds of naughty thoughts about fucking him. The next, she was sitting back in her chair, her mind trying to catch up with reality.

Krish disappeared from the room.

'Hey!' he said. The smack of a kiss 'What're you doing here?'

His voice sounded a little strained.

'I thought I'd surprise you, see how the meeting went,' said a perky female voice. 'What happened to your shirt?'

'Oh, um…Nothing.'

'It's covered in black streaks. You look like one of my reception kids after art.'

The visitor could only be the infamous Jess, and Francesca hit herself on the forehead. 'Shit,' she muttered to herself. Guilt rose in her. It would be awful if Jess thought something was going on between her and Krish. Francesca wanted him to be happy. He'd found somebody whom he loved, and she didn't want to ruin that for him. Maybe in fifteen years, Krish and Jess would get divorced after procreating a brood of children with Krish's infectious smile, and then Francesca could swoop in and have him, but right now was not that time.

Standing, Francesca grabbed a tissue from the box on Krish's side of the office, wiping any remaining tears and black make-up from her face as best she could without a mirror. She had no doubt that she didn't look her best—definitely not how she wanted to look when meeting Krish's girlfriend. As usual, fate had dealt her a shit hand.

The prick of tears stung her eyes, and she wiped them away. *Suck it up, Francesca*, she thought as she inhaled a shaky breath and stepped out of the room, the strain of her smile causing the corners of her mouth to quiver. She pressed her lips together.

As she entered the much sunnier main office, she had to blink a few times in the light. Wow, they made primary school teachers differently these days. All of hers had been older women with kind, wrinkled faces and thick glasses.

Jess stood only a few inches shorter than Krish, easily six feet tall without heels. Her puny jean shorts revealed long, toned legs ending in strappy Roman sandals. Blonde-streaked, curly hair hung to her buxom chest, and her blue eyes twinkled in the sunlight bouncing off the acrylic picture on the wall. On top, she wore a loose, off-the-shoulder, bohemian blouse in blue.

She wondered what Krish had told Jess about Francesca's sudden appearance in his life. Did Jess know that Francesca was his ex? Or had he fobbed her off as an old friend? Either way, Francesca was under no illusion as to why Jess had popped in: to check her out.

The way women do, Jess was taking her in, cataloguing Francesca's appearance. Jess' gaze flicked between Francesca's blotchy red face and Krish's black-marked shirt, and a brief widening of her blue eyes indicated that she knew exactly how the marks had gotten there. If it bothered her, she didn't let on. Francesca had to give her some credit. If she had walked in on her boyfriend covered in another woman's eye make-up, she would have lost her shit. Jess must be a really nice person. Exactly the type of woman Krish deserved.

'Oh, hey! You must be Francesca. I'm Jess,' she said, moving forward and holding out her tanned and tapered hand.

'Hi! I've heard so much about you,' Francesca said. All she knew was that Jess taught kids and could assemble Ikea furniture. Krish never talked about her.

'Same,' Jess said. She turned towards Krish, who was fidgeting with his sleeves, his attention shifting between the two of them. 'So how did the meeting go?'

'Um...good?' He slid his eyes towards Francesca and they linked gazes. They both laughed. It made her feel better; at least they weren't going to be awkward about what had almost happened. 'They're an interesting pair. They didn't flinch when I gave them the quote, which is good. They said they'd let us know by the end of the week.'

Jess smiled, revealing straight white teeth. 'That's great!' Looking at Francesca, she added, 'Lucky you were here, Fran, to do the video side of things. I'm sure they'll book with you.' She booped Krish on the nose.

Francesca's eyebrows raised. She hadn't realised Krish was a booping kind of guy. 'Yeah, really lucky,' she said, not trusting herself to say much more. Nobody usually called her Fran and lived.

'So, honey,' Jess addressed Krish, sidling closer to him, 'there's a craft stall in Camden Market that I really want to visit. Fancy coming with and a late lunch?'

Francesca felt like a third-wheel on this conversation. She pretended to remove a piece of dust from the corner of her eye.

'Um, sure. Let me just grab my things,' Krish said. Jess made herself at home on the grey sofa and started scrolling through her phone.

'Do you want a cup of tea, Jess?' Francesca asked, attempting to be friendly.

'No thanks. I'm good.'

Swivelling on her heel, Francesca excused herself to boil the kettle. She could use the caffeine right now, and she'd noticed earlier that their selection of tea blends had increased by 1000%. She may as well stay in the office and get some editing done.

Krish joined her at the kitchenette. The warmth of him standing next to her made the hairs on her arm stand on end, despite the muggy air. The kettle began to heat.

'You okay?' he asked under his breath.

'Yeah, fine.' She was anything but fine, but it would be best for everyone if Krish and Jess disappeared soon.

His hand rested on the countertop, inches from hers. 'We'll talk tomorrow, okay?'

She didn't dare look up at him as those stupid tears moistened her eyes again. She nodded and removed the boiling kettle from its base.

He paused for a second before exhaling loudly and pushing himself away from the counter. 'Right! All ready to go,' Francesca heard him say on the other side of the partition. 'See you later, Francesca!'

'Nice meeting you!' added Jess.

'Have fun at the market!' Francesca said, imitating the cheery note in Jess's voice.

They were all being so civil, when all Francesca really wanted to do was throw things. It was an infuriating dilemma: wanting Krish to be happy with another woman, glad that he'd found one that was kind like him, but hating it at the same time.

Human nature, eh?

She heard the door click behind her. To avoid destroying Krish's office, she walked over to the sofa, flopped onto it, shoved a pillow into her mouth, and screamed.

# 14

THE NEXT DAY, Krish didn't turn up at the office.

No text. Nothing. He just didn't show.

Francesca would be lying if she said she hadn't made more of an effort getting ready after her PT session that morning. A slash of eyeliner and a lick of mascara. All for nothing, it seemed.

Picking up her phone, she toyed with the idea of sending him a text. Her finger hovered over the keys, struggling to figure out what to say. 'Hey! Remember when I gave you a massive hard-on yesterday? See you soon?'

*Don't be an idiot, Francesca.* She put the phone down.

What was the point? He was probably still angry after her performance at the meeting, and he had every right to be. The chances of them booking that wedding were slim to none. It made her hate herself even more. Her and her stupid mouth and her even stupider hormones. She wiped at the wetness in her eyes.

By noon, she realised that he wasn't going to turn up and so she played heavy metal, loud, specifically because she knew he would hate it. Nothing like a bit of AC/DC's greatest hits to go with her mood. Mick popped up once, to ask if she could turn it down after complaints. He was so nice about it that she managed not to snap his head off, although it took a lot of self-control.

*Fuck the world.*

She replayed yesterday in her head like one of her video clips, over and over.

For a few moments, she had felt so safe in Krish's arms, like none of the bad stuff could get her. What would have happened if she'd looked up at him? If he'd curled around her the way he used to, lowering his lips to hers?

*Nope.* She shook her head. Not a good path to tread. Nothing happened, thank god. It would have ruined the fledgling friendship that they'd cultivated, despite their past. She didn't want to repay his kindness by blowing up his life.

That didn't stop her from playing the *What if...?* game, imagining what kissing him would have been like.

One thing that their near-miss did highlight was that she needed to get away soon. She had taken advantage of his generosity long enough. She frowned. She had enjoyed the week they'd spent working side by side, without her cricket bat in easy reach.

She flipped her notebook open and wrote TO DO at the top of a fresh sheet. *Get locks changed* was the first item on the list. She hadn't been back to her office since the robbery; she just couldn't face it. Honestly, she didn't have great memories of working there, but the price was right. If, by some miracle, they managed to book this wedding at Blenheim, then maybe she could afford a better office. It might be prudent to wait and see what happened before she called the locksmith. Yes, that seemed like a good idea. She drew a line through the first item on her TO DO list.

Next she wrote *Chase up file recovery.* She hadn't heard anything from the tech guy, the 'quick turnaround' promised on his website ringing false. She'd tried to phone him a few times, but it either rang out or was busy. No option to leave a message. Might as well try him now.

The phone rang a few times before a deep, annoyed voice answered. 'Yeah?'

'Hi,' she said, unsure. 'Is this Speedy Dan's File Recovery?'

'Yeah?'

'Oh, great.' She put on her sweetest enquiry voice. 'This is Francesca March. I dropped off my cards last Monday?'

'Hold on.' The shuffling of papers buzzed down the line. 'Yeah, I've got your job bag here.'

'Okay...well...have you managed to recover the files?' Her fingers drummed on the desk.

'Nah. Not yet.'

Her rage simmered. Other people's incompetence made her angry, especially when it affected her. Through gritted teeth, she managed to maintain a ghost of her over-friendly tone. 'Well, when will you be able to look at them?'

'Tomorrow. Maybe the day after.'

Her fingers ceased their drumming. She leaned forwards. 'You know, calling yourself "Speedy Dan" is false advertising. I need those files, like, *yesterday*.' Her wedding contracts all stated she'd deliver a highlights reel of the event to the couple within six weeks. The purpose was to tide them over until she could finish the big edit, which took months. She didn't like to let anyone down, and time was ticking.

'Don't get your knickers in a twist, love. They're in the pile.'

He really shouldn't have called her 'love'. If she were a cartoon character, the top of her head would have blown off, and she'd be emitting steam from her ears. 'You'll do the work TODAY or I'm going to come down there and personally insert those cards one by one up your incompetent anus. Do you understand me?'

Silence. Her mother often said, 'You can catch more flies with honey than with vinegar.' But actually that was a lie. Francesca had looked it up: flies also liked vinegar.

For a moment she thought he'd hung up on her, but then she heard his asthmatic wheeze.

Finally he said, 'I remember you. Short girl. Dark hair, yeah?'

'Yes?' she said, emphasising the S.

'Ha. I'd like to see you try. I'll get to them soon.' He hung up.

The only thing stopping her from throwing her phone was the cost of replacing it. She banged it against her forehead. Somehow, the video from the Bollywood dance class last Thursday triggered and started playing. Sighing, she watched it all the way through and realised that she hadn't practised the routine yet. Well, no time like the present. Restlessness had filled her body, and a bit of movement would do her good. She scrubbed to the beginning of the video and hit play.

KRISH DIDN'T WANT TO FACE FRANCESCA TODAY.

So he went for a three-hour jog instead. *Run, Krish, Run!* Whenever he had a problem to mull over, running helped him gain clarity.

What had happened—or almost happened yesterday—didn't mean anything. Of course she'd relaxed in his arms. She was upset. He was familiar. They'd once had strong feelings for each other, and those kinds of feelings never went away completely. Deep down in his heart, he even maintained affection for the first girlfriend he ever had, aged 14. Was he still attracted to Francesca? Yes. Was she still attracted to him? Maybe. Was he going to act on it? No.

In ten days, he was taking Jess to Paris. He'd bought first class tickets on the Eurostar and booked a room in a 5-star hotel. After dinner on the Saturday, they would take a private boat tour of the Seine, and when they finished at the Eiffel Tower, all lit up, he would get down on one knee. She would say yes, and they'd plan a perfect, wonderful wedding. Connor would be his best man. Grace would be a flower girl. His sister would insist on giving a speech, taking all the credit for introducing them. Krish would give a speech, too. Everyone would laugh the first time he referred to Jess as his wife.

In the meantime, he just wished his traitorous brain would stop imagining a scene that never happened. What if Jess hadn't walked in? What if he'd slid his fingers under Francesca's chin and lifted her lips towards his?

He ran faster to chase the images away, to punish himself. He broke out in a sweat.

Thankfully, Jess had been oblivious to the tension. As penance for his non-crime, they'd spent the afternoon perusing every single craft stall in Camden. He didn't realise Camden even *had* that many craft stalls. He'd always associated it more with punk rock and cheap clothes.

He passed a familiar birch-lined road, not far from the Knights' house. He hadn't gone there intentionally, but he might as well pop by. Anyway, he needed to speak with Stella about the Blenheim wedding, and he could take the opportunity to play with his goddaughter, despite being unsociably sweaty. Hopefully Grace wouldn't mind.

The electronic door bell echoed through the house, and he heard muffled movement inside. The door swung open, and Stella appeared, still dressed in her matching grey cotton pyjamas and holding Grace, who was slobbering all over a blue teething toy.

Stella looked tired, with dark circles under her eyes, but her face brightened when she saw Krish. 'Hey, you! What a great surprise! Come in, come in.' She eagerly grabbed his hand and pulled him into the house.

'I found myself in the area and thought I'd stop by...'

'I'm so glad you did. I feel like I haven't spoken to anybody in days.' She laughed a little manically. 'Forgive me if I gabble on too much.'

'Where's Connor?' He didn't have any shoots on. Krish still had access to Connor's work calendar on his phone in order to help out when needed.

'He's interviewing new assistants.'

'Whoops. Sorry.'

'Please. You couldn't work for him for the rest of your life. It's not like you're married to him.' She smiled, but it didn't reach her eyes.

'Has he had any luck?' The sooner Connor found a new assistant, the sooner he could stop feeling guilty.

'Not yet. Funnily enough, it's not easy to find another talented Oxford-educated ex-lawyer assistant. Tough shoes to fill. Drink?'

'Some water would be great, thanks.' They walked towards the kitchen at the back of the house. Grace kept her big grey eyes glued to him over Stella's shoulder. He made a silly face at her, and she chuckled.

'Are you training for something?' Stella asked.

'No, no.' *Just running* from *something,* he thought.

She put Grace down at her feet, and the toddler started crying. 'Gracie, just give mummy a minute. I need to get some water for Uncle Krish.' Then to him: 'Sorry. She's having real attachment issues right now. I think it's because she's teething. Not sleeping well either, which means I'm not sleeping well. Anyway, blah blah blah. How are the proposal plans coming? Not long now!' She handed him a full glass of chilly, filtered water.

'Good, good.'

'Nervous?'

*Terrified.* 'Nah. We've already talked about it. I'm pretty sure she'll say yes.'

He drank the water in one gulp and went to the fridge to fill it up again. The coffee cups on the drying rack brought back the memory of Francesca and that silly Ryan Gosling mug.

'I'm so happy for you, Krish. She's a great girl.'

'Who?'

'Jess!'

'Yes, sorry. Yes, she's great.' He pushed Ryan Gosling and Francesca out of his thoughts.

'How's the new business coming along? I checked out your website. Krish, it's truly stunning.'

After downing the second glass, he said, 'Things are starting to

happen. Possibly booked my first wedding. A big one. At Blenheim.'
*Or possibly not.*

Stella picked Grace back up and clamped the fussing child to her hip. Grace instantly settled.

'Actually,' he continued, 'that's sort of why I need to talk to you.'

'Oh? Sounds intriguing. What's up?' Grabbing a box of cereal from a cupboard with her free hand, she plonked it onto the counter, then opened a drawer to pull out a bowl. A spoon soon followed.

He watched Stella fumble with opening the cereal box, liberally distributing seeds and flakes on the marble countertop as she poured out the contents. 'Can I help you?'

'No, no, I'm fine.' She put the cereal away before shuffling to the fridge for the milk. He noticed that she had on some horrendous fluffy frog slippers. One handed, she twisted the cap off the milk container and poured it over her cereal.

'Well, it's a huge Indian wedding in three weekends' time, and I need a second shooter. Someone I can trust. Someone I know will capture exceptional pictures of the bride—she's beautiful, by the way —and who I wouldn't have to train up.'

'Okay. So who did you have in mind?'

'You.'


Stella froze. 'Me?' Her eyes went big.

'Yes. You.'

She hadn't shot a wedding since before Grace was born. 'Gosh, Krish, I don't know. I wouldn't want to mess this up for you.'

'Please, Stella. You're one of the most talented shooters I know. You'd do an amazing job.'

Although she loved spending time with Grace, she did miss the thrill of working. Shooting with Krish could be good fun, a convenient way to ease back into things and flex her muscle memory with her camera. And Indian weddings were always so colourful and enjoyable. Biting the inside of her lip, she decided to ask for more info before making a decision. 'How long is the job?'

'We'd leave on Friday morning and come back on Sunday. I've checked Connor's schedule and he doesn't have anything on those days.'

'Huh. That doesn't mean he hasn't planned anything. All he seems to do since we got back is work.' They'd only spent two evenings together chilling on the sofa and made love a handful of times (usually just before he went to sleep).

Krish suggested, 'Well, he can take Grace into the studio with him, if he needs to.'

'You do remember the studio, don't you? Equipment everywhere? It's not safe for a mobile child.' She pictured the long rolls of background paper standing in the corner tumbling onto her baby girl. No way.

'Well, he can work from home then. You watch her all the time. I'm sure he can handle a few days. Some father-daughter bonding time.'

It sounded so easy when he said it. Swallowing, she turned away from him to hide the sudden moisture in her eyes. Connor hadn't been spending a lot of time with Grace, either, leaving Stella to do all the childrearing. She understood that it was his name on the door, but she was keen to get back to work, too. Maybe somewhere with *her* name on the door. For some reason, she was having trouble broaching the subject.

Actually, if she was honest with herself, she knew the reason: fear. She was afraid to voice her worry, to suggest that he saw her dreams as inferior to his. What if he confirmed it? His actions since they'd got back already implied that he felt that way, but there was something scary and irrevocable about hearing him say it. Right now, she only *thought* that was what he believed. But if he said it out loud, then she'd *know*.

She willed the tears away and returned to her cereal. 'Did you talk to Connor about this?' Maybe they'd already discussed it. She took a bite of her late breakfast and felt milk dribble down her chin. She caught it on her sleeve, catching a whiff of her underarm at the same time. She really needed a shower, but Grace was not in a compliant mood.

'No, I thought I could just speak directly to you.' Krish watched her shovel more cereal into her mouth.

'Oh, you can! I mean, he's not my keeper or anything.' She just knew that Connor would push back when she asked him. No...when she *told* him.

'So you'll do it?'

She desperately wanted to say yes. 'I'll *think* about it. When will you know if you've got the job?'

'By the end of this week, they said.'

A yawn took her unawares, and she covered her mouth with the back of her hand. What must she look like to Krish? A slovenly mess, that's what.

'Stella...are you okay?' Krish was looking at her with his eyebrows drawn down and concern in his eyes.

'Yeah, I'm fine. I...' She stopped and hugged Grace closer to her. She had tried to talk to Connor about sharing the childcare last night after Grace was in bed, but one thing had led to another, and she'd ended up with his head between her thighs instead. Not that she was complaining, but sex seemed to be their only form of communication since they'd got back from their travels. He obviously thought a good orgasm would cure all her woes. 'I could just use a break from being mummy all the time. This house is starting to feel like a prison. Even just taking a shower seems impossible these days. The moment I put her down, she either cries or crawls. She won't even nap in her bed. She'll only nap when I'm pushing her in the pram. The minute I stop, she wakes up. I'm exhausted. And I have no mummy friends.' Might as well tell him everything.

'I'm sorry to hear that.' He stopped and considered her. 'Why don't I watch Grace for a bit? I could take her out in the pram...? Play with her here...? Whatever you need.'

The tears started rolling down her cheeks before she could stop them. 'You'd do that for me?'

'Of course. I'm her godfather, and we have lots of catching up to do.' He walked towards Stella with his hands outstretched, a clownish smile on his face as he said, 'Would you like that, Gracie? Shall we have a little play while mummy has a break?'

Grace scrunched up her face, but allowed him to take her. 'Yay, she likes you!' said Stella, elated. Perhaps it was the fact that both of the grown-ups in the room smelled like body odour. Maybe Grace associated stinky adults with comfort. Stella chuckled.

Before either Krish or Grace could change their mind, Stella rolled out the instructions. 'She has some toys on the floor in the living room. You need to watch her all the time because she's walking now and wants to explore. Be especially careful of the stairs because Connor hasn't put up the safety gates yet and before you know it, she'll be halfway up. Her pram is under the stairs. She should need a nap in about half an hour. Snacks are in the fridge. Is there anything else?' she said more to herself.

'I've got this,' said Krish. 'Let me distract her and you can make your escape.'

Was it bad that Stella wanted to laugh like she'd just gotten out of jail? And not just because she was having a break from Grace, although that was a big part of it. Krish had offered her more than just a helping hand; he'd offered her work, the prospect of feeling like herself again.

In that moment, she decided that, no matter what, she'd find a way to shoot that wedding. Connor would just have to live with it.

# 15

MID-MORNING THE NEXT DAY, Krish's ukulele case thumped against his leg as he rode the lift up to the office. After work, he would be attending a class with a world-renowned instructor from Hawaii. Krish was keen to learn some new chord progressions.

Yesterday, he'd spent hours playing with Grace so that Stella could have a break. She managed to have a nap and a shower, and she'd looked more like herself by the time he left. He wondered if Connor realised how much she was struggling. Should Krish say something? He wanted to tell Connor, but inserting himself into their problems was a bad idea.

Afterwards, he ran home, showered, and worked from his dining room table. But he couldn't avoid Francesca forever. Humiliation flooded through him again. What did she think about yesterday and that unexpected hard on? She probably felt embarrassed *for* him.

He had no idea what to say to her. Or even whether she wanted to talk about it. Knowing her, she'd probably pretend it never happened. He wasn't averse to that, although he also felt they should address it head on—no pun intended.

Also, he didn't know what state she'd be in when he arrived. Would she still be at maximum Carrie-level horror mode or simmering at an Emperor Commodus from *Gladiator*? When he thought about what she'd said to him on Sunday, it made him sad for her. The thought of being controlled by hormones like that. There must be something that could be done.

It occurred to him that he could blame his little incident on hormones, too. They seemed to give bodies a mind of their own.

The lift door opened. He squared his shoulders and twisted the handle. From the editing suite came the low buzz of computers powered on. He popped his head around the corner, but Francesca wasn't there. Then he caught a movement near the kitchenette.

Francesca had her green cordless headphones on, and she was dancing.

She had her back to him. He leaned against the edge of the partition wall, a smile pulling at his lips. He'd never seen her move like this before. They had gone to clubs a few times when they were together, but this was different.

Her hands and hips swayed back and forth to what seemed like a choreographed dance. She had chosen a short blue sundress today, and the fabric ruched up and down her thighs as her legs kicked and stepped. He couldn't hear the music, but he still enjoyed the show. Whatever the dance was, she had the steps down pat. It was effective.

In fact, part of him thought it was *too* effective. He moved the ukulele case in front of his cargo shorts. *Not again.*

Francesca whipped her hair around her head, and the kettle came to a full boil. Her headphones flew to the ground.

'Shit!' she said, retrieving them, which is when she noticed Krish and jumped. 'Christ on a bobsled!' She clutched her headphones against her chest. 'Didn't your mother teach you not to sneak up on people?'

'Sorry.' *Not sorry.* 'Great moves.' It was probably wrong to enjoy her discomfort, but he did anyway.

'Well, you're the one that told me to get a hobby.' She tucked the headphones around her neck and poured water into her mug. 'Cuppa?'

'Yeah, sure. And I'm in shock that you actually took my advice.'

'Very funny.' She swept her hand over the new tea selection. 'What do you fancy?'

'Just normal builder's tea.'

'Thank god. I can't even pronounce half of these.' Dousing a tea bag in water, she glanced at him. 'What's that thing between your legs?'

Krish's cheeks flushed and his eyes snapped downwards. 'My uke. I've got class tonight.'

'Ooh, play something for me!' She handed him his mug (the one with Ryan Gosling) and made for the sofa. 'Come on. I don't have all day.'

She seemed to be in good spirits. His shoulders relaxed, relieved that she didn't seem inclined to bite his head off today. Perhaps *not* talking about it was the best idea. 'Okay.' He sat down on the grey chair and put his case on the ground. The clasps snapped open, and he removed his instrument, a mahogany concert ukulele, shaped like a miniature guitar.

Settling it onto his lap, he tuned the four strings.

'It looks so tiny in your hands,' she said, leaning in for a closer look. He caught the scent of her shea butter shampoo, reminding him of the other day.

'Yeah...um. Anyway...' What should he play? He knew a few songs off by heart. Flicking through his mental index, he came upon one that he thought would be funny. He strummed the first few chords of *'Cecilia'* by Simon & Garfunkel. She'd always complained when he listened to them. Too folksy.

This time was no different. She groaned and flicked her eyes up, but didn't say anything, settling back onto the sofa to listen.

Plucking the notes and hitting the wood of the uke to mimic the song, he launched into the first lines. He had to keep his eyes on the strings so that he got his finger placements right.

Krish loved playing the ukulele. He found it freeing, in a way that the piano lessons his mother had forced on him as a child never did.

The uke was easy. The first time he picked it up, he'd been playing full songs within an hour. Whereas other instruments needed years of practice, the ukulele allowed him to express himself without the faff of worrying about technique.

As the words came out of his mouth, it dawned on him that he could have chosen a better song: singing about a woman who broke her boyfriend's heart and then went off with another man was probably a bad idea. He wondered again what had happened with Norman.

When the song ended, he smiled hesitantly and looked up to see her reaction.

*BLOODY HELL*. FRANCESCA HAD FORGOTTEN ABOUT KRISH'S TALENT FOR singing. They'd only ever done karaoke once, but the memory of it came flooding back. His voice, crooning Frank Sinatra. Her body, jumping onto his after he finished and having dirty, up-against-the-wall sex in the private karaoke room. Then afterwards, realising there was a security camera on the ceiling.

Her eyes slid to that little ukulele, so delicate in his big hands. Sort of like her and her petite frame...In hindsight, why the hell had she requested a song? She couldn't move. She was certain that she was sitting in a puddle of her own desire.

'What do you think? Am I ready for the big stage?' He rested his fingers on the body of the instrument, shaped like a woman's hips...

'Well, you know. Don't quit your day job or anything,' she said, hoping he wouldn't hear the huskiness in her voice.

'Does that mean you want another one?' he joked.

'*No*! I mean, no. I have to get on with my work. Deadlines...Um. Good job.'

She sprang off the sofa and dashed into the editing suite to put as much space between them as possible.

The rest of the day was agony.

She could feel his presence on the other side of the room,

working on his own pictures while she cut together footage of a wedding she didn't actually hate. She'd been having one of her good days and didn't have to fake being happy throughout the ceremony. In fact, she'd cried real tears during the vows. The bride and groom had a bittersweet story: she had been on the cusp of marrying somebody else when she realised she was in love with her childhood friend. They finally got together, had a baby, and decided to make it official. Then a few months later, he had a cycling accident and ended up paralysed from the waist down. He was in a wheelchair throughout the wedding. People like them reminded Francesca that others had it far worse than she did. Her pain was nothing special. She was nothing special.

Tears flowed freely down her face as she edited. She must have sobbed at some point because Krish put a box of tissues next to her and asked if she'd like some tea. She nodded and wiped her face. Thankfully she hadn't bothered with mascara that morning.

The end of the day finally rolled around. Well, end of the day for Krish. She would stay on for another few hours. Taking off her headphones, she cricked her head left and right, then stretched. She swivelled her chair around just as Krish switched off his computer.

'I'm going to head out. Get a quick bite before my class. You staying?'

'Of course,' she said.

'Okay.' He paused for a moment. 'Hey, I wanted to say—'

Whatever he was about to tell her got cut off by the insistent buzz of his mobile phone on the desk. He looked at the number and she watched his face tense.

'Is it them?'

'Yup.' He blew out a quick breath and answered. 'Krish Kapadia.'

She studied his features for some sort of reaction. A frown. A smile. A small creasing of his forehead. Anything.

'Yup...okay.'

Nothing. He gave nothing away.

He nodded. 'Right. Thank you for letting me know.'

Her stomach flipped and her eyes went wide. Krish hung up the phone.

She couldn't take it any longer. 'Well, what happened? Did we get it?'

'WE GOT IT!' he bellowed and started jumping up and down.

Bursting out of her chair, she copied him, both of them pogoing around the room. 'YES!' she yelled, punching the air. This was amazing news. It meant she could get a better office, pay the disk recovery guy, and so much more. Maybe she could take a holiday! Go to Greece and meet an unsuitable man and have no-strings-attached sex on the beach.

Their joyful frolicking brought them close to each other and, without thinking, she bounced straight into his embrace like she used to, her own arms wrapping around his neck and her legs hooking behind his back at the ankles. His large hands automatically cupped her bottom, the perfect fit.

The move surprised them both.

For a second they blinked at each other, their bodies coming to a stop while their chests continued to rise and fall.

And then their lips crashed together.

She kissed him like she hadn't kissed anyone for five years. She had forgotten about the firm feel of him and the way he always tasted of strawberries. As his tongue slid between her teeth, she dug her fingers into his hair and hauled him closer, bunching her hands into fists around the silken strands. He pulled back for a brief moment and nipped at her lip before continuing to explore her with his mouth.

Blood rushed to her head, making her dizzy with lust. Krish was kissing her. This wasn't happening in her imagination. She hadn't been making up the attraction. A delicious ache sprang to life below her belly.

Carrying her like she weighed nothing, he strode to the editing room door and kicked it closed. He pinned her against the smooth wood. Francesca moaned. With her dress bunched around her waist, she could feel his arousal straining at the thin material of her silk underwear. She pressed her body downwards and then back up again, enjoying the sensation of him sliding against the sensitive bundle of nerves between her legs.

His fingers dug into the skin under her thighs, tantalisingly close to where they met in the middle. She wondered if he could feel how slick she was, a flood that had started when he'd been singing that damned song on the ukulele.

She thumped her head back against the door and he dragged his mouth down her neck, sucking and nibbling as he went. She arched her back to offer her breasts through her cotton dress. His head dipped and he found her nipple with his teeth, biting down just hard enough to make her breath catch.

Memories of how sexually compatible they'd been flashed through her brain—how they both liked it a bit rough in the bedroom. She still had a pair of handcuffs they'd used in her drawer. They'd never been *Fifty Shades* level, but they had liked to play. Pleasure and pain, mixed together.

She shivered at the scratch of his new beard against her skin.

In the five years since they'd dated, she'd been with other men but never allowed the relationships to get emotional. The goal was always one thing: sex. Anything more than that was off the table. But kissing Krish now, she remembered how the mental connection sharpened her desire, stoked it into a white hot flame.

It wasn't the act that got her off; it was the person.

All she could focus on was how she wanted to undo his shorts, slip her pants to the side, and slide him into her. The urgent need to do just that had her holding onto him, one hand around his neck, the other reaching down towards his snaps.

The pling of the metal popping coincided with his hand folding over hers, stopping her.

'Francesca, we can't,' he said, his breath hot against her cheek. His kisses slowed and ceased. With one hand, he unhooked her feet from around his waist and lowered her to the floor.

For a moment, dizziness overwhelmed her, and she grabbed the fabric of his shirt to hold herself up. But then it passed, and the reality of the last five minutes—had it only been five minutes?—dampened her ardour. Her breath lost its haste. What the hell had they just been doing? What had the past five years been for, if not to keep her away from him? Ten days in the same office and she was panting for him like a horny puppy. She slipped out from the space between him and the door and went to her desk. Looking over her shoulder, she saw him lean his hands on the door, his head hanging low. Regret and guilt emanated from him.

She had two choices in front of her.

One. Acknowledge that they still had feelings for each other. Tell him the truth. Let him fully into her world and see if he might choose her. The thought of doing that made her heart beat faster with both hope and terror. She wasn't stupid. She knew what his answer would be.

Two. Push him away and do what she did best. Close herself off. Don't let anyone get close. Just survive.

She didn't even have to think about it.

'SHIT.' KRISH TURNED AND LEANED HIS BACK AGAINST THE DOOR, dropping his head into his hands. Big mistake. He could smell her on his fingers. He crossed his arms, tucking his hands away. What had they been doing? In the frenzy, he remembered biting her on the neck, sucking on her nipples. 'I'm sorry. I don't know what came over me.'

'Don't worry. It was a mistake.' She pulled her dress down over her hips. The red marks where his fingers had been disappeared under the fabric.

He should have had more self-control. This was his fault. 'I'm sorry. I—'

'Krish, stop apologising. I think we're grown up enough to know that it took two people.'

She'd jumped into his arms, and the feel of her and the smell of her...it had taken him back to a time when they were different people. Ever since he'd seen her at the wedding, some part of him had wanted to kiss her, to—

Suddenly the picture of the woman he planned to propose to next weekend swam into his vision. 'I'm going to have to tell Jess what happened.'

'No, you bloody well won't.'

'I won't lie to her.' He'd already lied by omission once by not giving her the full backstory on Francesca. He couldn't add a second untruth to the tally. That wasn't the kind of relationship he wanted to have.

Francesca turned and skewered him with her eyes. In them, he saw no warmth, just pure determination. 'Krish, what happened just now didn't mean anything. Have your feelings towards Jess changed in the past five minutes?'

Didn't mean anything? He'd been moments away from having sex with another woman. No, not just another woman: Francesca. 'No, of course not, but—'

'Then don't be selfish.' She took a step towards him. 'Telling her may make *you* feel better, but it'll only serve to make her feel bad when there's no need.' Poking the air between them with a sharp finger, she said, 'If you tell her about this, then I'm not going to shoot the Blenheim wedding with you.'

'You can't be serious.' He wouldn't be able to find anybody else to do the work that he trusted as much as he trusted Francesca. She knew that. Her words cut like a betrayal.

'I'm completely serious, so I'll be clear: I don't have feelings for you. Nothing is going to happen between you and me so...you'd only be fucking up your own life.'

Leave it to Francesca to put it so succinctly.

She tucked a strand of hair calmly behind her ear and stood up straight, as though the kiss—and everything after—really had meant nothing to her. 'I'll be out of your hair as soon as this wedding is done. We'll shoot it, and then you'll never have to see me again.'

His heart unexpectedly squeezed at the thought, even as he knew it would be for the best.

Francesca motioned for him to move. 'Anyway, get out of the way. I need the toilet and you've got a ukulele class to get to.'

Realising he was still blocking the door that they'd been pressed up against moments ago, he stepped aside and opened it. She walked out with her eyes fixed straight ahead, her scent brushing past as she walked by. He heard the click of the toilet door.

He froze with indecision. His heart wanted to go to Jess's flat right now and confess, scrub his conscience clean, tell her everything he'd kept back since Francesca reentered his life. That would be the right thing to do, and Krish always tried to do the right thing.

But if he did that, Francesca had threatened to walk out. Would she really do it? He knew she needed the money, so it would be against her own interests. But then again, he'd seen her act against her own interests before, the meeting with Ishani and Paramjeet being a prime example. Did he feel confident enough to call her bluff?

Then again, how would she even know if he told Jess? It wasn't like Francesca had a spy network; they didn't even have friends in common. Knowing himself, though, he'd probably tell her. Or Jess might come to the office to confront Francesca. He couldn't control Jess's reaction.

The Blenheim wedding was important. It could give his new business the big boost it needed to achieve early success. Nothing could stand in the way of that.

His thoughts in turmoil, his head counselled him to wait. Take a deep breath, go to his class, let his feelings settle, and then choose a course of action. Nothing good ever came from acting hastily—as that afternoon had already proven.

With a long sigh, he picked up his ukulele case and left.

## 16

Francesca stood in front of her old office building, its grey bulk blocking out the sun. The button outside still had *March Films* written in faded black Sharpie, reminding her that this was where she belonged.

A shiver ran up her spine. She'd forgotten how much she hated this place. Amazing how quickly she'd gotten comfortable at Krish's. It would be a wrench to return, but she had endured harder things in life. She could do it, even if it was just temporary until she found somewhere else.

She checked her watch. The locksmith should be here soon. An envelope containing the cash to pay his exorbitant emergency call-out fee lurked at the bottom of her bag, and she clutched it tighter. She made a mental note to ask Krish about her payment from the Blenheim job. In all the excitement, she'd forgotten to talk to him about her cut. She had just trusted him to make it a good number, at least five thousand for a two-day event. She needed the money soon. Her bank account was dangerously low, and she still had to pay the disk recovery man when he finally pulled his thumb out and did the work.

The office's rectangular windows leered down at her. Twelve

days had passed since she'd last been here. Twelve days since Krish rode in on his white horse and rescued her.

Thinking about him made her heart contract. She couldn't deny that she had enjoyed kissing him yesterday, and she would have happily gone further, despite it being a Very Bad Idea. Since she'd moved into the office, their attraction had hovered like a third person in the room, a tempting troublemaker whispering 'You know you want to!'

Perhaps it was better that they had got it out of their systems. It was done now. They could move on.

Except she wanted to do it again.

Her toes curled in her sandals as she thought about his mouth on hers, his fingers squeezing her arse, creeping closer to—

She fanned herself in the heat. Thank god he had a girlfriend. It was the only thing keeping her from ripping his clothes off. Well, that and her infertility. Francesca had to remind herself that Jess was a nice person. She was innocent in all this. Jess was Krish's future.

Even if she did seem a bit clingy with her twice daily phone calls and suspiciously cheery disposition.

Francesca pushed her jealousy aside. Jess was perfect for Krish.

In contrast, Francesca was broken. Francesca would bring only chaos to Krish's life. And of course, Francesca was a liar.

She remembered the first time she'd lied to Krish. It had slipped out when they were on their third date. By then, she knew that she liked him. *Really* liked him. They'd already slept together after the second date, unable to keep their hands off of each other. The chemistry between them sizzled. She'd never experienced anything so powerful before, a potent blend of his confidence, his kindness, the way he encouraged her and, of course, his gorgeous face and body. Even then, she'd thought he was too good for her.

Over dinner that night, the conversation had turned towards the future, as it often did at the beginning of potentially serious relationships, a dance new couples performed to see whether they had the same life goals.

For some reason, she recalled that he was eating soup. He passed the spoon through the thin broth as though fishing for something and asked, 'Do you see yourself getting married one day?'

'Is that a proposal?' she joked. 'Bit soon, don't you think?'

A slow smile spread across his face that did funny things to her. It was a smile that promised a future. He stirred his soup some more before moving on to the big question. 'What about kids? Where do you stand on having children?' She could tell from the way he casually dropped his eyes to his spoon that it was an important question.

This was the moment she'd look back on and wish she'd said something different. If she had just told him the truth, then he would have been able to walk away right then and there, before things got too heavy. Before they started spending almost every night together. Before they'd gone to Paris.

At that point in her life, her diagnosis was recent. She was still getting used to her ineffectual treatment; the knowledge that no cure existed; and what the doctor had imparted so indelicately about her fertility: *You'll never be able to have children.* Some small part of her hoped that he was wrong, that she could conceive. Coming from a big family, she had always wanted one, too—but one where she wasn't the black sheep. One where she felt loved unconditionally by her two kids, their dog, and her doting husband. Now that she was older and had spoken with others who lived with PCOS, endometriosis, and fibroids, she knew the chances were almost nonexistent. But back then, she hadn't quite accepted that yet.

'I definitely want them.' She fantasised about her children with Krish: his brown skin, her green eyes. His Lancelot complex. Her ferocity. They'd be amazing.

To be fair, she hadn't said *she* could have kids. But she wasn't dense. She knew he would have checked that conversation off his mental list and settled in to take their relationship to the next level. Destination: Married Bliss.

Which is exactly what he did. They got closer and closer, the sex more and more adventurous; their feelings deepened. She knew she was in love with him, but held back from saying it. In her heart, she knew that everything was based on a lie.

When they'd go walking in the park, he would see a child doing something cute and turn to her with a smile and that one-day-it'll-be-us sparkle in his eyes. She started having anxiety dreams.

Her subconscious created a million different ways for him to find out about her infertility and a million more ways for him to react, none of them good. She'd wake up covered in sweat. The insomnia she already suffered because of her conditions grew worse. Hiding it from him became a constant battle.

She couldn't face telling him the truth. To see the disappointment in his eyes, to see him withdraw his love from her...it would kill her. She'd already experienced his anger over and over in her nightmares. She couldn't handle it in real life.

So she invented Norman, the man who stole her away. The fictitious knife-wielding psycho who slashed her out of Krish's life. It seemed apt.

Walking away from him that day was the hardest thing she'd ever done. She couldn't even regret it, because she knew it was the right thing to do, but the sadness and sense of loss was crippling nonetheless. She continually reminded herself that now he could find somebody else to love, someone who could give him the whole perfect picture that he deserved.

That someone wasn't her.

After she'd left, her life went from bad to worse. She'd lost her dream job working for a documentary filmmaker because her symptoms made it hard for her to keep up with the hectic filming schedule. She never divulged her problems to her employer, not wanting to use them as an excuse. She'd been down that road before: unless she coughed up a wheelchair, her bosses always doubted her pain.

That's why she decided to turn to weddings, a job where she could set her own hours, work as little or as much as she wanted, spend most of her time at a desk, and still do something she loved: making films.

Except she didn't love it. Being constantly exposed to other people's happily-ever-afters only made her think of what she'd given up.

Five years later, she thought she'd finally moved on. She'd thought wrong.

When she relived the way she reacted to him yesterday, the fallow desire awoke in her blood; she knew she still harboured feelings for him.

How fucking depressing.

And that was why she was standing outside her dismal office, taking the first step to cut herself out of his life. Again.

As she searched for the key in her bag, she wondered what Krish was doing, how he felt about yesterday. Had he told Jess despite Francesca's objections? They both knew her threat to pull out of Blenheim was empty. She needed that wedding almost as much as he did. But she hoped that she had at least given him pause to think it through. There really was no reason to tell his girlfriend what happened. His future lay with her, not Francesca. She squeezed her eyes shut to keep the disappointment inside her.

She would survive. She always did.

Unfortunately, in the very heart of her body, since Krish came back into her life, a tiny light had ignited that wondered if survival was enough. A rebellious thought popped into her head: *don't you deserve more?*

Francesca squashed it down.

Inhaling deeply, she opened the main door and climbed the stairs, the familiar odour of ammonia and urine assaulting her. As usual, the hallway was deserted. She noted that somebody had spray painted more expletives on the wall, a rude but appropriate homecoming gift.

Studying the door in front of her, she noted with dismay that it looked worse than she remembered. The thieves' jemmies had left deep gouges along the edge. She ran her hand over the gashes and wondered if she could get away with filling them with putty.

Annoyingly her contract stated that she was responsible for fixing any damage from burglaries, one of those sneaky clauses that she'd missed when signing. And because she had skimped on her insurance—only covering her equipment and public liability (which all wedding venues required)—she couldn't expect any help from that quarter.

Her phone rang.

'I'm here,' said the locksmith when she answered.

'First floor,' she instructed him.

She heard him wheezing up the stairs and turned to see a rotund, sweaty grandpa huffing towards her, a black toolbox covered in children's stickers jangling at his side. He smiled at her, and she introduced herself.

Squinting at the door, he whistled. 'Wow, somebody did a job on that.'

'Yup.' She had eyes.

Putting his box on the ground, he wiped his hand down his leg. 'You'll need to get it replaced. No point changing the locks on that, sweetheart.'

'Can't we just fill it in with putty?'

He actually guffawed. 'Fill *what* in? I'm sorry to say there's no actual door where the locks need to go.'

In a fit of sudden rage, she kicked at the wall, forgetting she had sandals on. 'Fuck!' She limped around in a circle. Best to refrain from causing bodily harm to herself with the Blenheim job coming up.

Breathing deeply, she closed her eyes and asked, 'Okay, how much will it cost?'

'This is just a ballpark figure, but with parts and labour...' He scrunched up his face with concentration, considering the damage. '...I'd say about a grand?'

'Shit.' More bills she couldn't afford. Great. 'When can you do the work? Today?' She had some money she'd saved to pay taxes and to tide her over during the six weeks' recovery after her operation. She could dip into that.

'Ah, no. You'll need a builder for this.' The locksmith was looking at her with pity.

She sighed. 'Okay, well, thanks for coming out. Sorry it was for nothing.'

Shoving his hands into his pockets, he said, 'Well, not for *nothing*, sweetheart.'

'Sorry?'

'You still owe me.'

Suddenly he wasn't so grandpa-like. 'For what?'

'For coming out. You booked me for an emergency appointment. I came. You owe me 150 quid.'

Her head began to throb. Rational thought fled. Her face tingled from the rush of blood, and she could feel the cords on her neck growing taut. A small voice within her whimpered *Run!* to the locksmith, but the word never made it past her lips.

*Hulk, smash!!!*

'ARE YOU FUCKING KIDDING ME?' He took a step back from her. 'I've been *robbed*. A whole wedding's worth of files has gone *missing*. The bride's father did time for *hiding bodies*. There's a Teflon *rat* living in my flat that thinks poison pellets are snacks. My ex-boyfriend is dating a gorgeous fucking *Amazon*. And you want to charge me 150 quid for *not* fixing my locks?!'

'Yes?' he squeaked as he picked up his toolbox and backed towards the stairs.

Even as the words tumbled out of her mouth, she knew she was being unreasonable. He had a small business to run, just like her. And he was the only locksmith out of the five she'd called who had agreed to help her. 'FINE!' She reached into her bag and tossed the envelope of cash to him, which he caught clumsily. He scuttled to the stairs and disappeared around the corner. Francesca could hear the toolbox crashing against the front door in his haste to leave.

She started to cry, guilt making her wish she could rewind the past few minutes and try again. She didn't mean to scare him, but in PMS week, she had such trouble controlling her emotions. She rode an invisible roller coaster. Sometimes she felt like she should be given one of those buttons to wear, like women who were pregnant on the Tube. Instead of alerting people that she needed a seat, her button would let people know that she needed space and understanding.

She'd have to send a message to the locksmith apologising for her behaviour. She rested her back against the wall and did some of her breathing exercises.

Her phone rang again and she hoped it wasn't the locksmith, giving her a piece of his mind from a safe distance. SPEEDY DAN illuminated her screen.

Sliding down the wall into a squat, she answered. 'Hi, Dan.'

'Whassup.'

'Did you manage to get the files?' Her voice sounded sad and tired after her earlier outburst, even as hope flowered in her chest.

'Do you want the good news or the bad news?'

She sprang to her feet, automatically on alert. Nobody who started a conversation like that ever had anything positive to say. 'The good news?'

'Humph. Well, I only have bad news. Your cards are fucked.'

Her fingers squeezed the phone. 'What do you mean "fucked"?' She paced back and forth with her other hand on her forehead.

'I mean, I can't get your data. They'd all been triple formatted, and you shot some new footage on a couple of them...so, yeah. Fucked.'

'No, no, no.' This was a nightmare. She'd lost the data for the wedding of a bride whose father used to bury bodies for a living. He knew all the good hiding spots. Her contract stated that her indemnity was limited to the return of the fee originally paid, but she doubted Larry 'Chuckles' Bonneface would see it that way. She'd probably have to go into hiding.

'Sorry, Shorty,' Dan grunted, not sounding like he cared one way or the other.

A thought occurred to her. 'Is it possible you're just incompetent?'

The knob actually laughed. 'Love, I'm incompetent at many things, but data recovery ain't one of 'em.'

'This is the worst day,' she said and burst into sobs.

## 17

As THE CHEF massaged the chicken breasts, Krish moved his light stand a few inches to the left.

'Perfect,' said Connor, taking another test shot.

'I fucking hate raw chicken. Reminds me of my ex-wife,' said Roland Burr, celebrity chef and all around arsehole. He looked up at his audience of two with a crooked grin before picking up a knife and inserting the tip into the side of the slimy meat.

Behind the scenes, Krish and Connor shared an unamused look and got back to work.

Every year, Roland—or 'Chef' as he insisted on being called by everyone—hired Connor to refresh his personal branding shots, and because Connor hadn't yet found a new assistant, Krish came on the job. He would never leave Connor in the lurch.

Selfishly, today it also served the purpose of keeping him out of the office and away from Francesca—even though it meant he had to suffer through Chef's misogynistic banter. Krish hated it. Whatever kind of man Chef was, it was not the kind of man Krish had been raised to be.

Connor scrolled through the images on his computer. 'We've got this shot. Let's move onto the next set-up.'

Every year, Connor told Krish it would be the last year photographing Chef. He didn't like him either. But Connor seemed on a mission to work since he'd come back from his travels. So here they were.

Krish broke down the lights. He moved them to the foyer of the restaurant, next to the white head of a taxidermied cow. Krish's lip curled with distaste. Even a non-practicing Hindu like him had feelings about cows and took some offence at seeing them disrespected as wall decor. It reminded him of Gaston's pub in *Beauty and the Beast*: lots of wood and red brocade alongside antlers and stuffed animals. As the specialty of the restaurant was meat, he could understand the design choices, but Krish was a life-long vegetarian. His father wasn't religious, and they never went to the temple, even though they did observe some Hindu holidays—doing the fun things and leaving the ceremonial bits. But one thing his father had insisted on was that the whole family avoided meat, especially beef.

Chef wanted a photo of himself posing with the cow while holding a cleaver. Shutting away his aversion, Krish set up the lights to Connor's instructions. His thoughts drifted, as they had many times in the past two days, back to the afternoon he'd almost had sex with Francesca.

Time had not dulled the passion they sparked in each other. It was immediate and all-encompassing, overwhelming any rational thought. Not that he didn't have passion with Jess. Of course he did. But with Francesca, there was an edge to it. Something thrilling and free. With her, he'd been so much more adventurous in his lovemaking. With Jess, their sex life was athletic, but the one time he suggested tying her to the bed, she'd raised an eyebrow and shaken her head. He'd never suggested anything like that again.

But he also couldn't help feeling like he was missing out. Some of his favourite memories of making love with Francesca involved a little light bondage, on both sides. That delicious frustration that came from having his hands immobilised as Francesca licked and sucked and aroused when all he wanted to do was dig his fingers into her hair and pull her closer. Kissing Francesca had unlocked a Pandora's Box of memories.

He had great memories with Jess, too. She was kind and caring and dependable. Nobody could beat her for positivity. She always helped him to think through both the pros and cons of any idea when he became too focussed on just the pros. His entrepreneurial brain needed that mirror. And they had a good time together! They enjoyed running and chatting and he liked showing her new things that she'd never experienced in her somewhat sheltered upbringing. The smile of surprised delight on her face the first time she tried sushi still made him grin. No matter how good kissing Francesca had felt, she belonged in his past. His present and his future involved Jess, whom he loved.

After the Blenheim job, Francesca would be out of his life, so there was no point in worrying about it. Much as he hated to admit it, she was right; no reason to tell Jess and introduce problems into his relationship where none existed. Sometimes, it was kinder to keep a secret. Even if he did tell her, he knew Jess. He believed she would forgive him and he would work his arse off to make sure she knew he wanted *her* and only her. It was just one kiss, that he regretted. Unimportant in the bigger picture.

So why couldn't he stop thinking about it?

'Hey.'

Krish jumped. Connor was standing next to him.

He narrowed his eyes with concern. 'You okay? You seem a little distracted.'

'Sorry, boss. Just thinking about...you know...the Big Proposal next weekend.'

'Proposal?' interjected Chef, who was standing nearby, sharpening his cleaver on a whetstone. 'Don't fucking bother. Take it from me, mate. I have five ex-wives.'

Frankly, Krish was amazed that five women would marry this man. He must be filthy rich, because neither his personality nor his face was attractive.

'Well, come on then. What's your plan? How're you going to pop the question?' asked Chef.

How did the man make 'pop the question' sound so distasteful? The last person Krish wanted to share his plans with was Chef. He threw a panicked look at Connor, who took the hint and said, 'We're ready to shoot. Don't want to end up in overtime...'

Chef sniggered. 'Too right, you fucking cunt. You cost me a bloody fortune as it is.'

'But I'm worth it. Your ugly mug isn't the easiest subject.'

Connor added what he called 'The Twat Tax' to Chef's quote, trying to make it so expensive that he wouldn't book him, but Chef just kept coming back. Only someone as talented as Connor could make Chef's red, pockmarked face look good in photos. Krish was well aware of the extensive retouching required, having done most of it himself.

With an unattractive laugh-snort, Chef said, 'That's why I still have you around. Where do you want me to stand?'

While Connor directed Chef into position and started shooting, Krish's thoughts returned to Francesca. He wondered where she was right now and how she was feeling. Ever since she had told him about her problems with PMS, he worried about her. It really seemed to affect her life. He'd looked up PMS online so he could learn more about it. As the son of scientists, gaining knowledge was always his first port of call. Francesca would probably hate that he had researched it, but he didn't feel guilty for doing it. He still cared about her.

He'd found out that there was something called Premenstrual Dysphoric Disorder, which presented as an extreme form of PMS. When he looked over the symptoms, some of them seemed to dovetail with what she described: the drastic mood swings, acting out of character, irritability and anger...but he had no idea if she had some of the other symptoms, like the insomnia, lethargy, or breast tenderness.

When he'd had his mouth on her breasts the other day, she didn't seem to be in any pain. Quite the opposite.

Guilt scissored through him again and he sighed. All trails of thought led back to kissing Francesca. He really needed to stop thinking about it. Later, he'd go for another run as a form of therapy. And he'd stop cancelling plans with Jess. Two nights in a row, he had claimed to have too much work to do. He couldn't keep avoiding her. Hell, he was planning to propose to her in a week.

That gave him seven days to get his head in order. He'd stay away from Francesca. He could work from home. He'd just pop into the office tomorrow to get his drives, and then he could retouch at his kitchen table until they left for Paris on Friday morning. On Saturday night he would propose.

An intrusive thought sliced through the noise: was he ready for this? What if he postponed the proposal?

Yes, it would be a massive pain to reschedule everything, and he'd probably lose a lot of money, but was it fair to ask one woman to marry him when another was filling his senses?

Marriage was a big step.

His parents had provided a healthy model of the institution: they'd been married for over 35 years, and they never fought. If he had to describe their union, he would label it calm. And respectful.

He could have that with Jess. She symbolised stability and trust and longevity. That's what he wanted. It would be smooth sailing with someone like her. They'd get married. They'd have kids. They'd grow old.

Francesca, on the other hand...he imagined life with her would never be dull, but it would also never be smooth. Her changeable nature didn't presage a long and happy marriage, did it? This lust he felt for her...it was temporary. And there was still the niggling suspicion he had that she hadn't been 100% honest with him.

No, Jess was the right choice.

Once he had that ring on her finger, everything would fall into place. Decision made.

. . .

A FEW HOURS LATER, CONNOR SAID THE MAGIC WORDS: 'THAT'S A wrap.' Krish was glad to be getting out of there. He'd endured Chef's endless monologue comparing women unfavourably to various items of food. They'd had chocolate cake (tastes good but no good for you), artichokes (prickly on the outside, but hiding a delicious centre), and fish tacos. Krish didn't even want to think about that one. Again, Krish marvelled that Chef had been married five times. He hoped the women managed good divorce settlements.

Now that he had a plan of action regarding Francesca and Jess, the tension melted away. With renewed purpose, he packed up Connor's equipment and loaded it into the van. He circled back around the restaurant to make sure they hadn't left anything behind. At the rustic wooden bar, he found Connor flicking through the images on his laptop, Chef hovering over his shoulder.

'You're a fucking talented cunt,' Chef said to Connor. 'With that pretty face, I'd marry you myself if you weren't a bloke.'

'In that case, I've never been happier to be a man,' said Connor. Krish suspected he was not even half joking. Connor closed his computer, and Chef, chuckling, returned to his stainless steel kitchen.

Clocking Krish, Connor checked his watch and said, 'Let's get moving. Stella wants me home by seven. Says she wants to talk to me about something.'

Krish had a feeling he knew what it was, but just to play along, he said, 'Sounds serious.'

'I'm sure it's nothing. Even though she's been acting a little off lately.'

It was the perfect opening for Krish to share that he thought Stella was finding it hard being on her own all the time. He opened his mouth, but before he could say anything, Chef's voice interrupted, 'When my wives acted strange it was either because they found out I'd cheated on them again or it was that time of the month. Ha! You know what they say about women with PMS: they're like a soufflé...full of eggs, but if you beat her, she'll still go down.'

When Krish thought back to this moment, he couldn't recall how it happened. What Chef said hadn't even made sense.

But one second he was standing next to Connor, and the next, he was holding Chef by the lapel of his whites, his other arm pulled back and tensed for a swing. The only thing stopping him was Connor holding him back and hissing urgently, 'Krish! KRISH! Stand down.'

Red clouded his vision, and all he wanted to do was make Chef's ugly face even uglier. After a day of being forced to listen to Chef's anti-woman, anti-gay, anti-everything comments, Krish was at the end of his tether. And making fun of women with PMS hit too close to home for him to ignore.

Connor's voice slowly found its way through the angry haze. 'Krish, come on. Leave it.'

A flame of anger at Connor flared. How could he let this arsehole get away with the comments he'd made? Especially when they were directed at his wife?

Krish unfurled his hand from Chef's white uniform and unclenched his fist. He stepped back.

'What the fuck?' Chef protested, regaining his bravado as he shrugged his uniform back into place. 'Hit a nerve, did I? Somebody's got to put his big boy pants on.'

Connor pushed Krish further away from Chef. 'You okay?'

Not trusting himself to speak, Krish just nodded.

Squeezing Krish's shoulder, Connor turned to Chef.

The man's face was even redder than normal, the maze of broken veins on his nose practically glowing under the tungsten light of the bar. Pointing towards Krish, he said, 'Don't bring that pussy to any more of my shoots.'

Except he didn't say pussy, but another P word. Krish almost laughed at Chef's puerile attempt at insult: the age old fallback position of the feeble mind, resorting to racial slurs. *Nobody can hurt you without your permission*, Krish's father always said, quoting Gandhi.

Connor crowded closer to Chef and sniffed like he had smelled something bad. 'I don't know if your mother didn't love you or your father was a dick, or maybe both, but you seem to think your problems are everybody else's fault. No wonder your ex-wives divorced you. Frankly, I'm amazed they married you in the first place. You need therapy.' He turned and packed his computer into his bag. 'We're done here.'

Shock made Chef's mouth hang open and his beady eyes go wide. 'You fucking kidding me? You can't speak to me like that. Not with what I'm paying you.'

'You know what? Keep it. I don't want your money. And I'm deleting your photos.'

Krish didn't hide the smile that tore across his face at Connor's words, even as adrenaline coursed through his veins. Without a backward glance, he headed for the exit.

Once inside the van, Connor engaged the engine and backed out of the alley. Silence hung in the air as he waited for a space in the traffic to pull out.

Krish's hands still shook. He couldn't believe what he'd just done. It was unlike him to act so rash. With the all-encompassing rage coursing through him, he would have beaten Chef to a pulp if Connor hadn't stopped him. Normally level-headed, the sudden burst of anger confused him. His parents had always taught him the superiority of brains over brawn. What had triggered him to act that way?

Of course, he knew the answer.

Francesca.

'Are you okay? Want to talk about it?' asked Connor.

Krish looked out the window, his eyes unseeing. He had a lot of thinking to do. 'No.'

## 18

STELLA TOOK another sip of red wine as the front door clicked closed. The clock read 7:45PM. She'd asked Connor to be home by seven.

'Something smells gorgeous.' He entered the kitchen, dropping his bag on a stool. He sounded tired. She continued to stir the curry. It was based on a recipe they'd learned in India, his favourite. She also wore a short sundress they'd bought in Australia that showed off her legs.

He didn't apologise for his tardiness, but Stella bit her tongue. She had to keep her eyes on the prize tonight, which was breaking the news about leaving him in charge of their daughter for three days while she went to work with Krish.

Picking up the bottle of red, she poured a generous glass and handed it to him. 'Good shoot today?'

'Well, let's put it this way. I don't think I'll be photographing Chef anymore.' He took a long sip.

'Why? What happened?'

Leaning his hands on the island, he dipped his head and looked at her. 'He was spouting his usual misogynistic bullshit and… well…Krish almost beat the shit out of him.'

'What?!'

'Yeah, he lost it.' Connor sat on the stool next to his bag.

'That doesn't sound like Krish...'

'I know, but it happened. Honestly, he did me a favour. Chef is such a prick. Every time he books me, I think to myself it'll be the last time.'

Stella laughed. Thinking of Valentina, she said, 'At this rate, you aren't going to have any clients left.' She turned to Connor with a smile, but he was staring at something in the distance, his face serious.

'Earth to Connor...' Pushing away from the oven, she rotated his stool towards her and slotted between his legs. As she kissed him, his arms snaked around her waist, pulling her closer.

'Uh uh ah,' she said, drawing back from him and waving a finger. 'Dinner first.' She wasn't going to let him sabotage her plans.

'Actually, I'm starving. How's Grace?'

It would be nice if he asked how Stella was doing. 'She's asleep. We went to the zoo today. Again.'

'Yeah, I know. I saw the pic you posted on Instagram.'

It was a really cute picture of Grace at the penguin pool. A penguin had swum up to them, and she'd reached out a hand, as though she could touch the bird through the glass. It was just a simple snap on her phone, but the image felt full of natural wonder mixed with the joy of childhood.

Connor caught Stella's chin with his finger and stroked the cleft. 'I thought we'd agreed we wouldn't put pics of Grace online.'

Stella pulled back from him in surprise, and his hand returned to her waist. 'Oh, sorry! It's mostly just the back of her head, so I thought it would be okay. I'll take it down.' Her cheeks heated.

'It's nothing big...' He kissed her on the forehead, like he had already forgiven her.

'Yeah, yeah. I know. Don't worry. I said I'll take it down.' She pushed herself away from him and picked up her phone. Within moments, the photo was gone from her feed. A rush of sadness washed through her. She'd loved that photo. Now she wouldn't be able to look at it without remembering this exchange instead of the event itself.

Returning to the oven, she tried to shake off the awkwardness. Of course they'd agreed not to post pics of Grace, but she really wasn't identifiable. *He's overreacting*, she thought. Even so, the reprimand stung.

However, she had bigger fish to fry tonight. She couldn't get distracted. Slapping a smile on her face, she offered another morsel of cute Grace information from her day to get him back on side. 'She said *Zebba*.'

'She's a genius.' He plucked an olive out of a bowl.

'And her walking is coming on. She keeps crawling out of her pram.' Stella didn't want to tell him the whole story. She had been taking a break for a minute, sitting on a bench with the sun on her face and her eyes closed. When Stella opened her eyes a few moments later, she had the shock of her life. Grace had managed to sneak out of her pushchair and toddle away.

Thankfully one of the zoo employees brought Grace back, babbling away in toddler-speak and blissfully unaware of the heart attack she'd almost given Stella. Bad mother vibes clung to her—a feeling she was getting overly familiar with. She stirred the curry and pushed the feeling away.

The wedding. She needed to concentrate on that. When Krish called her the other day to tell her it was happening, she confirmed immediately that she was on board. One way or another, she would be there, even if the thought of leaving Grace for three days filled her with anxiety. But she had to get over it. She needed to do this job for her own sanity.

It wasn't like Connor couldn't handle it. While travelling, they had both taken equal responsibility caring for Grace. Only since they'd returned had it reverted to Stella's full-time job. Connor went happily to work every day, and she'd become, well, her *own* mother, Angela.

That was not what she wanted. This job with Krish might help to rebalance things.

She spooned the curry and rice into bowls and told Connor to follow her into the dining room.

'Hmmm. The fancy china. Is it a special occasion?' he asked as they settled into their seats.

Stella lit the candles on the table. 'No. I just wanted to spend some time with you. I feel like we haven't talked properly since we got back.'

'This looks delicious.' Connor leaned forward and inhaled deeply.

'Remember the night we had this in Jaipur? The little old lady with the eyepatch and the—'

'—gangster monkey on her shoulder?'

They both laughed and took a bite, recoiling at the same time. It was too hot to eat.

Taking a sip of wine to cool her tongue, she said, 'So what do you think was up with Krish?'

'No idea. He didn't want to talk about it, but in hindsight, he was a little quiet all day. I should send him a quick text and check he's okay.'

Stella thought about the nights when Connor came home and she'd been quiet. He noticed more about his assistant than he did about his wife. She clenched her jaw, but carried on. 'Any luck finding a replacement for him?'

'Some good options, I think. It's the interview process I hate. I'll know within a minute whether I'm interested, but I'll still have to see out the full half an hour. Anyway, I've got them lined up for next weekend.'

Sitting up straight, Stella frowned. 'As in, not this Saturday, but next Saturday?'

'Yeah. Why? Is that a problem?'

No time like the present...

Squaring her shoulders, she said, 'Connor, I'm going to be away that day. In fact, I'm going to be away for three days. I'm assisting Krish at a big wedding in Oxfordshire.'

'When did this happen? He didn't mention anything to me.' He crossed his arms.

She did the same. 'I asked him not to. I wanted to talk to you about it myself.'

'How long have you known?'

'Since Tuesday.'

He threw his hands up in the air. 'And you're just telling me now?'

'Well, to be fair, I haven't really seen that much of you.'

'You could have called...?'

'I wanted to talk to you face-to-face.'

He rubbed his temples with his fingers. 'What about Grace? Are your parents coming down?'

'No. I thought you could do it. You know, being her father and everything.' She gave him a hard look.

Shaking his head, he said, 'I've got two days of back-to-back interviews at the studio on Friday and Saturday. I can't bring her with me.'

'I'm sure you'll figure something out.'

'How am I supposed to "figure something out"?' He used his fingers as air quotes, which really pissed her off.

Her voice rising, she said, 'I don't know. Call your brother. Maybe he can help.'

'You want to leave our one-year-old with my brother, who has no experience with children?'

'He's an internationally celebrated barrister. I'm sure he could figure out how to watch Grace.'

'Unlikely. He's probably not even in the country.'

Stella could feel her temper escalating. He wasn't even trying to meet her halfway on this. 'I've got a great idea. Why don't you cancel your appointments and spend some time with your daughter? Get some stuff done around the house? Put up the stair gates. Take her to the zoo. Experience the wonder of a Peppa Pig marathon.'

'This is really inconvenient.' He leaned his head back against the chair and closed his eyes.

'Well, I'm sorry if my life is inconvenient to you, but I'm doing it.'

Eyes snapping open, he said, 'That's not what I meant.'

'What did you mean, then?'

He was quiet for a moment, his forehead tensed in thought. 'What is this about? Are you worried about money?'

She threw up her hands. 'No, Connor, it's not about the bloody money. It's about me. I want to go back to work, too. I'm sick and tired of you assuming that I'm going to do all the childcare until she goes to nursery. It's still months away. And she has two parents. I'm miserable by myself all day. Don't get me wrong; I love Grace, but I'm lonely. And it's not the most exciting age. I just need a little help.' Tears edged her voice, and her eyes pleaded with him to understand.

That silenced him. She could tell that he was trying to formulate a response, so she ground her teeth to prevent herself from filling the conversational void. What if he told her that his job was more important than hers because his name was above the door? Would he do that? She knew when she married him that he had a big ego, but she'd come to think of Connor Knight Photography as *their* business. What if he didn't?

Grace squeaked on the monitor, and Stella held her breath until Grace settled again. Connor exhaled, as though he'd held his breath, too. The moment would have been funny if so much wasn't riding on it.

Lowering his voice, Connor said, 'I'm sorry. I didn't realise.'

'Yeah, I know.' Hot tears pressed behind her eyelids.

'Go ahead and do the shoot.'

She turned her head away from him as a tear slid down her cheek. 'Thanks for your permission.'

'Stella, I'm trying to work with you here. I just said I'll watch her.'

He dropped his head into his hands. 'I'll try to be around more. It's just...since we got back, I've...I don't know. Felt like I need to play catch up. Make sure people haven't forgotten me. Earn loads of money so I can take my foot off the brake while I work on my fashion portfolio. Also I don't have anything recent to enter into this season's awards cycle, and I need to shoot some new material. I keep trying to organise spec shoots, get a creative team together, but I don't have the time to do that and run the business because I don't have Krish or you right now.'

Reaching out, she placed her hand on his arm. 'You *do* have me. I can help. I know how you feel about nannies...' As the son of a diplomat, he'd been raised exclusively by nursemaids after his mother died. He repeated often that he didn't want that for Grace. '...but maybe we should get one just for the next few months until Grace goes to nursery. I want to do some shoots, too. I've got so many ideas—'

He pushed his chair back and beckoned to her with his finger. 'Come here.'

She took a last sip of wine, got up, and straddled his lap.

'I love you,' he said. 'Just in case I haven't told you enough lately.'

'I know.' She smiled, reassured that they had finally communicated with each other. For the first time in ages, she believed everything would be okay. They were a team again. She could trust him to have her back.

She didn't know why she held onto things so long, waiting until they built up into a bomb blast, instead of bringing them up when they first occurred to her.

Digging her hands into his dark hair, she lowered her lips down to his. He grabbed her head and deepened the kiss while she pressed her breasts against his chest, letting him know exactly what she wanted. Connor growled.

He moved his hands to her bottom and stood up in one smooth motion, carrying her to the stairs. Setting her down on the carpeted steps, he looked at her, a devilish gleam in his eye as he pushed her sundress up around her waist and relieved her of her underwear.

By the time they got back to the curry, it was cold.

## 19

Francesca nailed the dance.

As the students went over the moves from the previous week, Francesca hit every hip thrust and hair swing. When it came to the new choreography, she managed not to look as hopeless as last time. She glowed when Jaiveer approached afterwards and commented on her improvement.

'You surprised me, Goldie. I thought you'd be a one-class wonder. Glad you came back.'

The next morning, she walked to the office from her flat, choosing the extra exercise over the expediency of public transport to delay the possibility of seeing Krish. Her heart beat faster, and not just because of the pace she set herself. A sense of dread hung over her. Mostly, she hoped he wouldn't be there. The less they saw of each other in the run up to the Blenheim wedding, the better. But a small part of her just wanted to breathe the same air as him.

Stopping, she fought the urge to slap her own face. *Not the right attitude, March.*

She had a wedding to shoot that weekend and needed to get her equipment. A visit to the office couldn't be avoided. Next week, she planned to work from home, doing the tedious but necessary task of copying the drives under her bed so that she had a second set of back-ups.

Thinking about it made her groan. She still hadn't figured out what to say to the gangster bride whose footage had been stolen in the robbery. Sweat began to bead between her breasts. She could only deal with one thing at a time. Right now, she had to focus on putting together a team for the Blenheim wedding two weeks from now. So far, calls to her contacts had returned nothing. She needed a second shooter and a drone operator, but everybody she knew was busy.

All she seemed to have were problems. The sudden urge to call her dad frothed up inside her, much to her surprise. She quickly dismissed it; he would just share some pointless anecdote about rowing that wouldn't give her any answers and then go on about how hot it was in Spain. No, she'd deal with her problems all by herself, as per usual.

'Hey, Mick,' she said to the security guard, now reading *The Tibetan Book of Living and Dying*. Basically, Mick got paid to read. Nice life.

She rode the lift up, jiggled her key in the lock until it turned, and went inside the office. The lights were all off, the room quiet. Great. Krish wasn't there. She walked into the editing suite.

'Hey.'

'Christ on roller-blades.' She grabbed at her neck and tried to ignore the jolt of happiness that pierced her, forcing the corners of her lips to curl down and not up. 'KRISH! Are you trying to give me a heart attack? Why are you sitting in the dark?' She dropped her bag onto her chair.

To be fair it wasn't completely dark. His screen was on, casting him in a white ethereal glow. Saint Krish. Francesca flicked on the light switch.

'Sorry. I didn't know if you'd be in today.' His chair creaked as he leaned back and crossed his arms.

Perching on her desk, Francesca mirrored his body language,

arms scissored across her chest like a security gate. 'I just came by to pick up some stuff. I'll be out of your hair soon. And I'm going to work from home next week, so…you know...'

His pointer finger drew circles on his desk. 'I'm away from Friday—'

'On a job?'

'No.' He looked up and held her gaze. 'I'm going to Paris. With Jess. We've had it planned for a while.'

'Oh.' Francesca studied her feet as they lapsed into mutual silence.

Paris. He was taking Jess to Paris. The very place Krish and Francesca had gone many years ago. A flare of jealousy tinged with anger rose within her, and she squeezed her hands into fists. Paris was *theirs*. It had been the best holiday of her life. Sitting next to the Seine, eating warm baguettes and drinking wine out of paper cups. Joining in an impromptu dance party on the steps of the Sacre Coeur. Making love in the rickety budget hotel that claimed to have once hosted Albert Camus.

She hated that her heart was thumping at 200bpm. She hated that she wanted to cross the room and stake her prior claim on him. She hated that her lips were aching to kiss him.

Her arms still crossed, she dug her nails into the side of her ribs, reminding herself of the reasons she couldn't do any of those things. She pressed her nails harder, until she was surely drawing blood.

Pain. That's who she was. That's what she would bring to Krish's life. The pain of her infertility. The pain of her conditions. The pain of loving somebody who was broken. She couldn't do that to him.

'We need to talk,' he said.

Her head whipped up. Those were the same words she'd said to him when she'd broken up with him. *Talking* was the last thing she wanted to do. 'I'm in a hurry, Krish—'

'This won't take long.' He stood up and walked towards her. How was it that she could feel the air between them as it displaced, pushed aside by the pressure of his body? She gulped in a deep breath, and he stopped a couple feet in front of her.

Her instinct was to move away, but her limbs wouldn't comply. Body tense, she attempted to arrange her features into a bland expression of disinterest, as though she was the Duchess of I Don't Fucking Care. 'Okay. Talk.'

'Francesca, what do you want from your life?'

The question took her unawares. She didn't know what she'd expected, but that wasn't it.

What was he asking? Did he want a list of goals? Did he want her to say she hoped to get back to documentary film making one day? Tell him that she dreamed of making a film that exposed the way women were often medically gaslit when talking about their own bodies? How she wanted to create a documentary so powerful it helped increase the funding to research historically female conditions?

Or was he asking about love? Did he want to know that she pined for a normal life? For someone to care about her? To wake up one morning miraculously cured?

She couldn't say any of that to him.

What did she want from her life?

'To survive it,' she said, lifting her chin defiantly.

His warm brown eyes warmed with concern. 'Do you think that's a healthy goal?'

Anger bubbled inside of her. Easy for him to ask; he, who had his life all worked out, everything falling into place. She really shouldn't be having these kinds of conversations in PMS week. She said, 'I don't have the luxury of thinking about the future. I have too much on my plate right now.'

'Are you happy?'

Why was he asking these questions? What she wanted to say was: 'No, I'm not happy, Krish. I'm in a bad place and I could really use your help. The disk man couldn't retrieve the files from my cards and I have to call the bride to tell her I've lost all her wedding footage and refund her money. I'm afraid her dad is going to have me whacked. I want to get out of the lease for my old office, but I have to replace the door and locks first which costs a lot of money. I'm worried about the Blenheim job: that I won't be able to find a team, that I'm going to be in pain that weekend, that I'll let you down, which I do not want to do. And on top of it all, I think I still have feelings for you.'

What she did say was: 'Are you my therapist?' He raised an eyebrow, daring her to answer his question. 'I think happiness is for people with money and options. I have neither.'

She couldn't stand the look in his eyes. It was dangerously close to pity and she didn't want that. It only made her feel even worse.

Sighing, he said, 'I wish you were kinder to yourself.' He reached out to tuck a strand of hair behind her ear. Her breath caught, and her skin burned where he touched her. 'I wish you could see yourself the way that I see you.'

She blinked at him, and her heart crawled into her throat. That's how it felt: like her heart was on the verge of escaping her mouth and exploding all over the room. She took a deep breath and tried to regain some equilibrium. Staring at his chest, against her better judgment she asked, 'How do *you* see me, then?'

Shoving his hands into the pockets of his shorts, he huffed a laugh. 'Well, you're strong and stubborn, crazily talented, and funny...but I also feel like you're a...a geode: hard on the outside and hiding something beautiful. Like you're afraid. But what are you scared of?'

A *geode?* She'd been compared to many things in her life, but that was a new one. Right now, she was scared that if she opened her mouth, all her secrets would come pouring out. She would lay them on the floor in front of him, a sordid smorgasbord of her inner demons, and let him fight them for her, one by one.

Instead, she grabbed her bag and stepped towards the door. 'I have to go—'

His hand wrapped around her wrist. 'Wait. Francesca, what is this between us? There's something still there. You can't deny it.'

'I can deny it. I will deny it.' She turned and faced him. 'Krish, yes. I know there's an attraction. But that's all it is. We used to have really, *really* awesome sex, and I guess our bodies remember that. But that's it. Sexual attraction.' She had to end this now. She puffed up her chest, going in for the kill. 'I broke up with you once because I didn't see a future for us. And I still don't.' Looking hard into his eyes, she said, 'I don't want you, Krish.' He winced and her heart seized. She couldn't stop there. She needed to hammer in the nail once and for all. 'Besides I'm...I'm dating somebody else.' It had worked once and it could work again. She needed to create a new Norman. Who would this one be? John McClane from *Die Hard*? Ethan Hunt from *Mission Impossible*? Then it came to her. 'His name is Jaiveer. He's a choreographer.'

Inside, she flinched. The disbelieving look on his face made her physically hurt. Her Bollywood dance instructor had been the first person that jumped to mind, and now she had to run with it.

'You never mentioned that.'

'Why would I? We're not *friends*, you and me.' She sneered the word and hated herself for it. 'It's not like I'm going to have a gossip with you around the water cooler. And in case you've forgotten, you're dating Jess.'

Perfect, beautiful Jess with the golden hair and clear skin. Practically a poster child for health and fertility and a much better match than a mess like Francesca would ever be. Jess or the Mess? No contest. 'Go back to your *girlfriend*. Because *this*—' She wafted her hand between the two of them. '—it's never going to happen.'


KRISH WATCHED AS FRANCESCA STALKED OUT OF THE ROOM AND turned towards the equipment storage, closing the door behind her.

That had not gone at all as he had planned. He had hoped she might open up to him, tell him how she was really feeling for once, but all he'd gotten for his efforts was her hard shell. She flipped from passionate to distant in a milli-second; he could practically see her building her wall, brick by brick. And then—surprise surprise—the final brick: a new boyfriend, appearing out of the blue. He didn't push it, even though he didn't believe it either. Something wasn't adding up.

Since leaving Connor's studio after their job yesterday, he had done a lot of thinking. At home he laid in bed, awake half the night, lost in thought. He'd even forgotten to eat, which meant this was really serious.

After almost punching Chef, Krish had to acknowledge one glaring fact: he had feelings for Francesca. Strong feelings. Feelings that made him want to get into fights for her like some sort of modern-day Rocky Balboa. But Krish had never been in a fistfight in his life, despite having the muscles for it. Only one explanation made sense for his knee-jerk reaction yesterday: he loved Francesca.

But he also loved Jess. How could he love two women at the same time?

Jess and Francesca were polar opposites. Jess was like water and Francesca...well, she was definitely fire. Jess was calm and caring, the kind of woman that would be a solid life partner, mother, and lover. Somebody he could count on.

But Francesca...she was *exciting*. She was passionate, vivid, colourful, and magnetic. He had so much in common with her and she made him laugh in a way that Jess never did. Living with Francesca would be a never-ending roller coaster. Years ago, he vaguely remembered talking to her about what she wanted from life...Marriage? Children?...but he couldn't remember what she'd said. Maybe he should find out.

However, the big question he had was: what did *he* want in his life? Water or fire?

Of course, the whole thing was moot if she didn't want to be with him, so he set himself the task of asking her.

And he had.

But Francesca did not want him. Whatever her reasons, she'd made that abundantly clear.

He watched her leave the room and decided not to follow, even as a fist squeezed his heart.

AS HE ESCAPED THE BUILDING FOR SOME FRESH AIR, HIS PHONE RANG. His sister's name flashed across the screen. Krish didn't really want to speak with her right now, but they had plans to confirm.

'Hey, hey, Little! How ya doin'?' Her bright, husky voice pierced through his sadness.

He cleared his throat so he could match her tone and hide how lost he felt. 'Hey, Big. All good. You?'

'Looking forward to dinner with you and Jess tomorrow night. '

He closed his eyes and ran his free hand through his hair. It would be the first time he saw Jess since his kiss with Francesca. 'Yeah, what time do you want us? What should we bring?'

'Just yourselves. Seven o'clock?'

'Great.'

She paused for a second. 'What's wrong? You sound off.'

Ankita knew him too well. Normally he would confide in her, but she loathed Francesca. If she were on fire, Ankita wouldn't even consider the possibility of giving Francesca a glass of water. Part of him thought Ankita had also felt betrayed when Francesca walked away. His sister and his ex-girlfriend had grown close in the time they'd dated, but Ankita saw things in black and white. Once Francesca left, Ankita's affection had turned cold overnight.

His sister had helped him through the breakup. She'd seen first-hand how devastated he'd been. Telling her that he had considered leaving Jess for Francesca was not an option; she'd give birth on the spot. 'I'm just tired,' he said and changed the subject to something that would distract her. 'How's the Belly Bean?'

'I cannot *wait* to get her out of me. I'm counting the days. Forty to go. This little sucker better not be late.' For the baby's sake, Krish also hoped she didn't screw up her new mum's schedule. Ankita liked to be in control of things.

Remembering that he had some good news, he said, 'Did I tell you? I booked a big wedding. A huge two-day Indian affair.'

'Really? That's fabulous! Anyone I know?' Ankita worked in entertainment law and seemed to know everybody. She was always dropping names, but now it was his turn to drop one.

'I don't think so. Well, maybe. It's Vashney Oberoi's son.'

'The big Bollywood director. Well, hot damn, Little!'

'I know. Between you and me, his son's a bit of a prick, but it'll be great for my portfolio.'

She made a pfff noise. 'He's not that bad.'

'What? Do you know him?' Krish wouldn't be surprised.

'No, sorry, I mean, I'm *sure* he's not that bad. Anyway, gotta go. I have another call. See you tomorrow!' And she hung up.

His conversations with Ankita were always sharp and fast. Time was literally money in her job, where every second of her day had to be logged against a client. It was one of the things he'd hated about being a lawyer.

He pocketed his phone and looked up towards his office windows. Francesca hadn't even responded when he said goodbye. In a way, he was glad she'd been so direct with him. There was no question now about what he should do.

Francesca was not an option and it wasn't fair to Jess that he was dithering like this when she had no idea. So no more dithering. Jess and he had two years of building a solid relationship under their belts. He knew Jess. He trusted Jess. He would dedicate himself 100% to making her happy and giving her the marriage she deserved. They had all the ingredients they needed to make a long, stable life together. He would continue with his plan to propose.

Despite this clarity, something niggled at him. A thought that had started as a seed and had grown steadily with every step he took, and the thought was this: Jaiveer the Choreographer seemed awfully convenient. She'd never mentioned a boyfriend, and suddenly one appeared, as though by magic.

Which led him on the short journey to wondering about *Fucking Norman*. Had he been real? Or had Francesca created these imaginary boyfriends as a way to push Krish away?

And if that was the case, that left another big question.

*Why?*

## 20

THE OFFICE WAS quiet without Krish.

Not just quiet. Empty. A void. A man cave without its man. A joyless cell.

Francesca lay her head on the back of her chair and twirled around in a full circle. Then she did it again. And again. Her hot water bottle flew off her lap, landing with a thud on the floor.

It had been a long and lonely week. First there was the wedding she'd shot on Saturday. Tedious, predictable, and clichéd in every way. Thankfully, her pain from the endometriosis and fibroids waited until Sunday morning to make its monthly appearance. She'd spent Monday through Wednesday tucked up in bed with ibuprofen and a bottle of vodka, trying to stay off the co-codamol in case she needed it for the Blenheim job. While her hard drives had copied over to a second back-up, she edited on her tiny laptop screen. She hated working on just one screen when she was used to having all her menus, timelines, and film clips spread out over three. Having everything scrunched together in such a minuscule space gave her a headache, on top of everything else.

But it was worth it to avoid Krish.

She glanced over towards his empty workstation.

Right now he would be packing for his trip, printing out his tickets, checking the weather for the weekend. 'Bon bloody voyage,' she said as she spun again.

In her head, she heard Krish's voice: *I wish you could see yourself the way that I see you. You're strong and stubborn, crazily talented, and funny.*

Her cheeks glowed red. He had the crazy part right. The more she tried not to think about it, the more his words echoed around her skull. She wanted to find pleasure in them, but instead they had the opposite effect. She visualised her thoughts as a game of Whack-a-Mole: every time one popped up, she'd bash its head in with a hammer. Her heart hardened just a little bit more. She had done the right thing.

And then there was his other question: *What are you scared of?*

'Everything,' she said aloud to the empty room.

A sharp pain in her side made her wince. She picked up her hot water bottle, a pink rubber thing shaped like a penis. It had a big smile on its willy face, a party favour from her sister Donna's hen party a few years ago. Francesca pressed it to her abdomen.

In some good news, she had found the team members she needed for the wedding at Blenheim: David, a drone operator whose portfolio looked amazing, came highly recommended to her by an old film school colleague, and her second shooter was Wally, who she'd worked with a long time ago. Finally, things were falling into place. They both had their own kit, too, which took a load off her mind, even though she could actually afford to buy whatever they needed now. In fact, she could afford to have the door at her old office replaced, too.

She was rich. Well...comparatively.

After their talk, she had sent Krish a very professional and impersonal email to ask when she'd get paid and what number to put on her invoice. The number he sent back in his equally professional and impersonal email made her eyes water, making her realise she really *hadn't* been charging enough for her services. Thank god Krish wasn't in the room when she found out, because she might have jumped him again.

The money was in her account the next day. Keen to get out of his office, she had already engaged a builder to do the work on her door next week. After the Blenheim wedding, she'd move out. She'd sit tight for the final month of her lease and then find somewhere nicer to work.

Another spasm pierced her body, and she bent over, praying for it to pass. After a few minutes, she relaxed as the pain eased.

A buzzer rang in the other room, and Francesca got up cautiously to investigate, bringing Hot Willy with her. The noise sounded again. She realised it was some sort of doorbell. She hadn't realised they had one.

Opening the door, she found a slim, beautiful redhead woman with a stylish grey pram, whom she vaguely recognised, but couldn't place.

'Hello,' the visitor said. 'You must be Francesca. Krish has told me all about you.'

Francesca cleared her throat. What exactly had he told her? That statement contained a lot of possibilities. With a suspicious edge, she said, 'And you are...?'

'Sorry! I'm Stella Knight. And this is Grace.' She motioned towards the chubby, pink-cheeked cherub sleeping in the pram. She pushed it forward, indicating that Francesca should step aside.

Without thinking, Francesca did, her attention focused on the baby as it was wheeled past her. She didn't have a lot of opportunities to be close to children, and when she was, she experienced a strange push and pull. The push was the fact that they served as a reminder of the type of family she'd never have. The pull was curiosity. What did it feel like to hold one? What did it feel like to breastfeed? What was she missing?

She shook her head and refocused on her guest. So this was the famous Stella. In a way, she reminded Francesca of Jess: tall and lithe with perfect skin. Wife and mother material.

Francesca knew she should be welcoming and friendly to Stella, who was a good friend of Krish's and would be working the Blenheim job with them. On the other hand, she just wanted to be alone.

'Krish isn't here,' Francesca said, holding the door open to encourage Stella back through it.

'I'll wait.' She parked the pram in the corner and engaged the brake.

'Actually, he's off today. Getting ready for his big trip to Paris. With his girlfriend.' The more Francesca said it, the more she'd accept that Krish was with someone else.

Surprised, Stella stopped short. 'Oh! I thought he would be in today. I should have called to check before popping in, but I was in the area. Never mind. Gives us a chance to get acquainted.' She leaned over to check on Grace. 'She should stay down for at least another hour. Fingers crossed.'

God, Francesca hoped they wouldn't be staying for a whole hour. It took so much energy for her to hide her pain from others. Almost on cue, a cramp scissored across her abdomen and she cleared her throat to hide the grimace of discomfort. She pressed Hot Willy to her middle. Stella's eyes dipped down towards the pink water bottle, and her perfect lips curved in a sympathetic smile. 'That time of the month, eh? I know what that's like.'

*No, you fucking don't*, thought Francesca. She hated it when other women got pally over periods, like they all experienced them equally the same. Most of them had *no idea*.

Stella twisted her wedding ring on her finger, then fanned herself with her hand. 'It's so *hot* out today.'

Great. Now they were going to have a lovely chat about the weather. How very British. 'Yeah. Roasting.'

Awkward silence.

Francesca filled her cheeks with air like a chipmunk and blew it out slowly. She wasn't sure how much more obvious she could be that she wanted her guest to leave. Stella was either thick, which

Francesca doubted, or so desperate for company that anybody would do.

'I'm very thirsty,' Stella said. 'Shall we have a cup of tea?'

'Fine.' With an audible sigh, Francesca tossed Hot Willy onto the sofa. She trudged towards the kitchenette, Stella's light footsteps following behind her.

Reaching up into the cupboard on her tippy toes, Francesca pulled down the tea presentation box and dropped it onto the counter with a thud. Motioning towards it, she said, 'Choose your poison,' and filled the kettle.

'Oooh! I'll have this one.' Stella handed over something Chinese. 'I first had this when I was in Singapore.' She paused. 'We just got back from travelling around the world for six months. Krish probably told you.'

'He mentioned it. Bet it was a blast,' she said flatly. The last thing Francesca could handle right now was one of those tell-me-what-you-did-on-your-travels conversations that people who had gone away pressed on people who hadn't. Francesca would have loved to take a break from her life and go traipsing across the earth, but unfortunately, the one thing she most wanted to escape would come with her.

Another pain in her side made her fumble the Fornasetti mug in her hands. The kettle started to bubble. Francesca hoped it wouldn't wake up Grace and make her scream, but Stella didn't seem concerned.

'So...' she began, as though looking for something to talk about, 'Krish hasn't sent me the schedule yet. Do you know what it is?'

This, Francesca could handle. 'The Mehndi party is on the Friday. You know...where they do the henna designs on their hands and stuff—'

'I've shot loads of Indian weddings. I love Mehndi Night. Are they doing a Sangeet, too?'

'Yes.' A Sangeet was a sort of dance party where each of the families showed off their moves. Francesca remembered the famous Sangeet scene in *Kabhi Khushi Kabhie Gham*.

'Blenheim is such a stunning venue.'

Of course, Stella would have shot there with Connor and Krish. 'I've never been.'

The kettle boiled, and Francesca filled Stella's cup, automatically adding some cold water from the tap to cool it down. She didn't want to wait for the hot tea to reach drinking temperature, thereby extending the visit. 'Milk and sugar?'

'Just black, thanks.' Stella took the mug and went to sit on the sofa. Francesca gritted her teeth and made herself the same drink. Might as well try some of these funky teas before she went back to her own hole-in-the-wall office.

Kicking off her shoes and folding her legs underneath her body, Stella got comfortable on the sofa—a little *too* comfortable for Francesca's liking. She wasn't used to this level of aggressive friendliness from a stranger. Stella had the air of someone who got on with others easily and couldn't understand that not everybody wanted to be her bosom buddy.

Sometimes, Francesca wished she had a little more of that quality. Her walls were built so high that people naturally sensed her lack of emotional availability. She sat in the grey armchair, making sure to keep Hot Willy on her stomach. Another stab of pain. She breathed deeply in and out, pretending to blow on her tea.

'I'm a bit nervous,' Stella confessed. 'I haven't shot a wedding since before I had Grace, so almost a year and a half. May I?' She indicated the show albums on the coffee table, and Francesca nodded.

'I'm sure it's like riding a bicycle.' Francesca sipped the tea and almost spit it out. It tasted like smoky water. How could Stella drink this stuff? While her guest looked through the albums, Francesca let the liquid slide from her mouth back into the mug.

'When did Krish say we're leaving?' Stella asked, as she turned a page and drank her tea, seeming to enjoy the disgusting brew.

Francesca had to admire her determination to keep the conversation going. In an alternate universe, Francesca was sure she'd love to get to know Stella, but not here and not now. 'Um...he's renting a mini-van to drive the whole team up together. Leaving from here on Friday morning, I believe. Going straight to the Mehndi Party.'

'Ah. And where are we staying?'

'Some bed and breakfast nearby.'

Another awkward silence descended, and Francesca wished she could hide her discomfort in sips of tea, but she wasn't putting that shit in her mouth again.

Finally, Stella said, 'Gosh, it's so exciting, isn't it?'

'Yes. It'll be a great wedding.'

'No, sorry. I meant Krish and Jess.'

Francesca blinked. What did she mean?

While still casually flipping through the album, Stella said, 'Paris is so gorgeous. So many memorable places to propose.'

PROPOSE? Krish hadn't mentioned anything about that. Her stomach clenched like she'd been punched and she spilled the tea onto her bare legs. 'Shit.' She got up and ran over to the kitchenette for a cloth, glad that the false wall hid her from Stella's view.

Unaware of Francesca's distress, Stella continued, 'My husband, Connor, asked me to marry him in Madrid...'

Blood roared in Francesca's ears, making it impossible to hear more. Krish was *proposing* to Jess—even worse, in *Paris*...where a lock with 'K&F' on it had once adorned the Pont des Artes before the government removed them all; where Krish and Francesca had asked a passing tourist to photograph them kissing in front of the Wall of Love; where Krish had said those three words she both yearned for and dreaded. She'd wanted to say them, too, but the words stuck in her throat, blocked by her own wall of reasons.

She leaned over and put her hands on her knees, sucking air in and out of her lungs like she had just finished a long race. Forgotten streaks of brown tea ran down her legs, pooling in her sandals.

Krish—*her* Krish—was getting engaged.

She didn't know why it shocked her so much. She'd told him that she didn't want him, so he was free to do as he pleased. As he'd said, this weekend had been scheduled a while ago. When Francesca revealed that she 'had a boyfriend', he was probably relieved. It meant he could carry on with his precious plans, get on with building his perfect life with his perfectly fertile baby goddess.

So why did it feel like her heart was going to detonate at any second?

'I wonder who Krish will ask to photograph his wedding,' Stella said from the sofa, and this time Francesca couldn't hold back a loud sob.

Suddenly, Stella was there. 'Are you okay?' She stood near the partition wall, her forehead riddled with concern.

Only then did Francesca realise that she had hot, salty tears pouring down her face. 'Yep. Fine.'

'Shit,' Stella said before moving closer and putting her hand on Francesca's back, rubbing in a circular motion like a mother comforting her child. 'Your period pains must be something else.'

Still bent over with her hands on her knees, Francesca nodded, happy to let Stella think that was the cause of her anguish.

'Can I get you anything?'

This time Francesca shook her head no.

Stella continued to rub her back. It actually felt quite nice. Her own mother had never done this, not being the touchy-feely type.

Continuing on her new favourite subject, Stella said, 'Krish photographed my wedding.' She obviously thought that blathering on about weddings might take Francesca's mind off the pain. She wished Stella would just be quiet, but, no. She continued: 'Although I have to wonder if he might ask Connor to be his best man. Jess will make a beautiful bride, don't you think?'

A picture of Jess standing next to Krish at the altar filled Francesca's mind. She couldn't take it anymore. Her shoulders shook as the sobs returned.

Stella's hand stilled for a moment before resuming its circular motion. 'Oh. I see. This isn't about your period, is it?'

Francesca's cheeks burned with shame. Standing so that Stella's hand fell away, she grabbed a piece of paper towel and wiped it across her face, her snot leaving slug trails. Attractive. 'What else could it be about?' She blew her nose.

Tilting her head to the side, Stella crumpled her eyebrows in sympathy. 'Do you...want to talk about it?'

For a moment, Francesca considered it. How nice it would be to let the words pour out of her mouth, to share the burden of her feelings with somebody else—even better, somebody who knew Krish well and might have some insight into what she should do.

But that just wasn't her. She didn't know Stella, and she certainly didn't trust her.

Francesca wanted nothing more than to turn off the lights, curl up on the sofa, clutch Hot Willy, and disappear from life for a while. 'Nope. Thanks. I probably just need to lie down.'

'No problem. We'll go. Sorry to have taken up so much of your time.' Stella washed out her mug and put it on the drying rack before heading to the pram and unlocking the foot-break.

The spilt tea made Francesca's sandals squelch as she followed Stella to the door. Holding it open, she said, 'I guess I'll see you next week.'

Stella stopped just outside of the door and turned. She paused as though deciding whether to say something. 'I understand that you don't want to talk about this with me. I mean, who am I to you? You don't know me. But...I hope you have somebody to talk to. I know from experience that it can help.' She pressed her lips together and offered a thin smile before turning to call the lift.

As soon as they disappeared into the lift, Francesca closed the door and slumped against it, the tears sliding unchecked down her cheeks.

*Bloody bollocks and whangers.*

Krish was well and truly lost to her, and now she couldn't help but wonder: had she just made the biggest mistake of her life?

# 21

THAT NIGHT, Francesca attacked the dance.

She had moved through the shock phase of grief and entered the anger phase. Everything she saw suffused her with rage: small dogs in prams, people walking too slowly in front of her, couples. Especially the couples. They were just showing off with their hand-holding and kissing and pavement hogging.

Why had Krish come back into her life? She'd been doing perfectly well without him. And why did he ask her all those questions before he left?

And why didn't he tell her he was proposing to Jess?

And why couldn't she just tell him the truth? Why had she been saddled with this body? She hated it. It was weak and she hated weakness.

*But weren't you being weak by not telling Krish your secret, so he could make his own decision?* She screamed and groaned at the same time, the sound of a wounded animal.

Sacrificing one of her saved-up co-codamol days, she took a couple of the white pills before heading downstairs to her Bollywood class. She needed physical activity. She didn't care if she was getting the moves right, she just wanted to dance like nobody was watching.

But somebody was watching. 'You have such passion tonight!' said Jaiveer fervently during the break. She noticed a touch of something new in his gaze. Was it respect…or lust?

Inside, pent up energy mingled with her heightened emotions, as if she could explode at any second and take out half the block. She needed release. Any release.

Maybe she could find some release with Jaiveer. She'd already told Krish they were dating, so why not make it a reality?

After the class, she stretched until everyone else had left except him.

'Good work tonight,' he said as he packed up his bag. 'You're really improving.'

Shaking her hair free of its ponytail and draping herself on the ballet bars next to him, she said, 'It helps that you're such a great teacher.'

He raised an eyebrow on his thin, hawkish face. 'There are some things that can't be taught, and tonight you had it. There was fire inside of you.' His faint Mumbai accent was quite sexy.

With a flirtatious look, she asked, 'Fancy a drink? I know a place around the corner…'

He slung his bag over his shoulder and considered her with warm brown eyes. He did have nice eyes. Darker than Krish's. 'I suppose I could have one drink,' he said.

'Great.' She undraped herself from the ballet bar and closed the distance between them, making sure to put some extra wiggle in her hips. She ran a single finger down his muscled, dancer's chest and tilted her head to the side. 'Or we could skip the drink? I live just upstairs…' She caught her bottom lip in her teeth and gave him her best under-the-lid Lauren Bacall look.

Francesca knew that she was attractive. She never struggled getting a man on the rare occasions when she wanted one. And tonight, she wanted one. She couldn't be alone with her feelings.

Jaiveer glanced down at her hand, which was stroking his chest. He smiled. 'I'm flattered, but you're not really my type. I'm gay.'

'Oh, fuck.' She dropped her hand and took a step back, cheeks going hot. 'I'm sorry.'

'It's fine. Happens all the time.' He winked.

She swallowed, finding the next words hard to admit. She struggled with being needy. 'I-I just could really use a friend right now.'

She didn't have a lot of friends. Any, actually. She had colleagues and acquaintances, people she had worked or studied with. But no bosom buddies. Nobody she could pick up the phone and call when she needed bad advice and certainly nobody who would start a sentence with, 'Girlfriend! Let me tell you what you need to do.' When she saw close female friends in TV shows and films, they seemed like complete works of fiction. Did women really go to the spa together for mani/pedis? Did they really go out to brunch every Sunday? Not in her experience. Perhaps that was why she never could get into *Sex and the City*. It seemed like a fairytale. When your whole world revolves around hiding yourself and putting up walls, it was hard to grow your social circle.

Sometimes Francesca felt like a piece of paper, folded and folded and folded until it was as small as it could be. That made it easier to slip between the cracks of other people's lives.

Jaiveer considered her with a soft gaze. Was it pity? No, she realised with relief: it was concern. There was a huge difference. 'Shall we go get that drink, then?'

Stella's words came back to her, advising her to talk with somebody. Well, Jaiveer was somebody. 'Okay,' she said. 'That would be nice.'

TEN MINUTES LATER THEY WERE SITTING IN A QUIET CORNER OF A local pub, the kind that still had a carpeted floor and upholstered chairs that remembered the days when people could smoke indoors. Thankfully, it wasn't too busy, so they found a table easily.

Both of them looked completely out of place in the old man's pub, her in her sweaty lycra and Jaiveer in his stylish black ensemble. She swirled her vodka and tonic and wondered how normal people embarked on conversations about their personal lives. She didn't have a lot of experience with these kinds of chats. Should she just start talking? Ask him about himself first? Comment on the weather?

'So, Goldie. Tell me what's going on.'

Ah, that would do it. She took a deep breath and began, 'Well, um, it all started five years ago...'

Jaiveer leaned forward and listened to the whole story, beginning with the day she met Krish at a bar in London, to their discussion about children and her secret infertility, to the breakup, fast-forwarding to present day.

'And now he's off to Paris tomorrow to propose to his new girl-friend because I'm too broken to give him what he wants!' Tears spilled down her cheeks. Shifting his chair closer to hers, Jaiveer put an arm around her, a gesture that normally, Francesca would find awkward, but now that Jaiveer knew all her baggage, it was sort of nice.

'I wouldn't call yourself broken.'

'I *am*. I'm infertile...'

'So? Last time I checked, having children is not the only thing a woman's good for.'

'I know, but he wants them. Krish does. And I can't give them to him.' A fresh wave of tears exploded out of her. Even though she'd known this information for years, the wound unexpectedly reopened. Her petite shoulders shook with renewed vigour and tears mingled with an uncomfortable amount of snot. She wondered what the etiquette was for wiping her nose on someone else's shoulder while being comforted.

As though reading her thoughts, Jaiveer produced a tissue from somewhere and handed it over. 'You know there are other ways to have a family? This is the 21<sup>st</sup> century. I mean, is he in love with you or your womb?'

'He's not in love with me at all.'

Jaiveer tsk-tsked. 'Really? Why do you think he asked you those questions last week? Not because he doesn't *care*—'

'There's a big difference between caring, like, for a friend, and *love*—'

'—So you told him that *I'm* your boyfriend,' Jaiveer laughed, 'and took away his chance to make up his own mind. Does that sound about right?'

'I already know who he would choose: the tall blonde baby goddess.' She sniffled.

'You don't know that.'

Francesca shrugged. 'Well now you know all my messy secrets.'

'Yes, I do.' He paused. 'And I call bullshit.'

'What? Seriously?' She drew away from him and crossed her arms. She suddenly remembered why she didn't like sharing her feelings.

'What are you hiding from?' he asked.

Francesca opened her mouth to reply and then shut it. It was a good question. Getting hurt? The thought of emotional turmoil on top of her physical pain just seemed like the proverbial straw to break the camel's back. As long as she could keep the two separated, she was safe. Her shoulders slumped. 'I don't think I'm strong enough to deal with getting my heart broken on top of my other pain. So I build walls.'

'Goldie, you haven't built a wall…you've built a cage.'

Francesca blinked as Jaiveer's words sunk in. A cage…she'd never looked at it that way before. Tears filled her eyes as the truth of it sunk in. She'd been keeping herself emotionally numb for so long that all this feeling was firing through her body like an electric shock. 'It's how I survive. You have no idea what it's like to live with chronic pain. It limits my options.'

'You're right. I can't even imagine what you deal with. But

survival has become your cage. At what point do you cross over from *surviving* to *thriving*?'

For once, she had nothing to say. It seemed so obvious, now that he put it like that.

'So in the meantime, you can't let it hold you back. You need to live. Otherwise, you'll wake up one day and find out life has passed you by and you're some old *budhiya* with saggy *babbes* and loads of regrets.'

'That's bleak.'

Was this what friend chats were always like? They were brutal. No wonder why she had avoided them.

With a shaky sigh, Francesca leaned back and closed her eyes. Jaiveer was right. She'd thought that if she could just keep herself sealed off until the time was right, she'd eventually get her happily ever after. And when she did, everything would magically fall into place. She'd find some wonderful divorced father, marry him, and that would be the beginning of her life. Or maybe she'd find a guy who didn't want kids. She knew they existed—except that didn't solve the fact that *she* wanted a family.

But what if, by the time she found this unicorn of a man, she was too emotionally stunted to fall in love? What if the numbness became permanent? What if there was no wonderful life partner available at the moment she was ready for one? Maybe she needed to stop only looking after her body and start looking after her soul, too. But that begged the question: was she already too late? 'What should I do about Krish?'

'Well, do you love him?'

Her bottom lip trembled. She knew the answer; she did love Krish. Kind, talented, funny Krish who made her body light up like a bonfire whenever he came near her. 'But he's engaged.'

Jaiveer shrugged. 'If you don't tell him, if you let him marry somebody else without knowing all the facts, you will regret it for the rest of your life. And regret eats at a person from the inside.'

She laughed without mirth. The thought of confessing her secrets to Krish made her nauseous. 'It's not that easy, you know. What would you suggest I do? Shall I go gyrate in a field and sing a song confessing my devotion? Real life isn't like a Bollywood film.'

'Your life isn't like a Bollywood film because you are making that choice. Don't you deserve a happy ending?'

AFTER HER DRINK WITH JAIVEER, FRANCESCA WALKED HOME WITH A spring in her step. She loved Krish. Maybe there was still a chance for them. Maybe all she had to do was tell him, and he would break off his engagement, and choose her. She just need to get out of her own way. A strange, warm light spread through her chest, and at first, she had trouble identifying what it was.

Hope. It was hope.

But on the other hand, Krish had already made his choice and it wasn't her. The hopeful light sputtered. Telling him her truth wouldn't magically change his mind, plus she couldn't just steamroller his life because it benefited her.

Jess was the star of his Bollywood film. It was she who would be gyrating in a field, singing about her love for the hero, a village of chipper children dancing behind her and praising her potential fecundity.

Francesca frowned. It had taken her exactly 134 steps from the pub to her flat to find herself exactly back where she'd started.

She unlocked her door with a heavy heart. Krish couldn't possibly love her. She had manufactured his feelings for her in her head. New tears arrived. Her resolve evaporated. She threw her keys onto the kitchen counter with a sob.

How would he propose? The question wouldn't leave her alone. She crawled into bed with her laptop and searched 'Best Places to Propose in Paris', studying each spot and imagining Krish getting down on one knee, Jess's magnificent head of blonde curls glinting triumphantly in the French sun.

The mound of tissues next to Francesca grew with each burst of emotion. Gone was the hope from earlier, replaced by an undulating flow of wet, hot sadness. Between her gut and her heart, Francesca struggled to get a handle on herself. In one crazy moment, she even picked up her phone to text him:

**Please don't do it. Fx**

It took two seconds to erase, horrified that her thumb might accidentally press send.

She contemplated texting Jaiveer, who had given her his number, and asking him to meet her for coffee in the morning. She liked his vision of her future and wanted him to paint the picture for her again. But she couldn't do that. Their friendship was still new, and she didn't want to be too needy too fast. He was probably busy anyway. At drinks, he'd said as much. Since he won his Fanfare award, his choreography services were more and more in demand. In fact, he would probably have to stop running the Thursday class soon. Another thing that made her sad.

But the idea of being alone with her thoughts that night filled her with panic, knowing that in the morning Krish would be zipping off to Paris with Jess.

Maybe she should call her sister? Donna was the only member of her family who seemed interested in having a relationship with Francesca. She always sent an invitation to her house for Christmas, but Francesca had never gone, worried that the invite was extended out of pity rather than sisterly love. Francesca couldn't shake the belief that her family collectively viewed her as a mild inconvenience. The problem child. The unhappy accident. When Francesca had started complaining about her 'lady issues', they labeled it as 'histrionics' and nicknamed her 'Hurricane Francesca'; but as it turned out, there *had* actually been something wrong with her. She wasn't 'lazy' or 'looking for attention' or 'being over-dramatic'. She was verifiably in pain.

It was partially because of them that she'd become so good at hiding it.

So, no, she wouldn't call her sister.

That left...nobody.

She blew her nose loudly and added another tissue to the pile. Her life was a real mess.

A dull throb in her abdomen added to her pile of woe. She pushed her laptop aside and picked up Hot Willy off the floor, trudging to the kitchen to fill the kettle. As she waited for it to boil, a familiar scratching sound came from under the sink.

King Rat.

Her body tensed and she reached for the cupboard handle, then stopped.

Francesca bit her lip. How did he keep avoiding the poison? It was almost like he knew that the little blue pellets weren't good for him. Like it or not, King Rat was a survivor, just like her. She laughed mirthlessly, as she realised that she had more in common with a rodent than with most people.

She filled Hot Willy with boiled water and clutched it to her stomach as she slid onto the floor next to the cupboard. Slowly, she prised open the door and peaked inside. King Rat stood on his haunches, his paws wrapped around the end of a celery stick from her compost bin. The little white diamond on his forehead froze as his glassy obsidian eyes stared at Francesca.

Sitting back, she attempted not to scare him. They studied each other for a long moment, neither moving a muscle. Eventually deciding that the food was worth the danger, he began cautiously chewing again.

'Hey,' she said.

*Hey!* She imagined his reply.

'You enjoying that?' She wrinkled her nose at the slimy green stick.

*Don't judge. One man's trash is another man's treasure.*

'True.' Why did the rat sound like a Jewish grandfather from Brooklyn? 'So tell me, what's it like being a rat?'

*It's okay. Can't complain.*

'Really? Even though everybody hates you?'

*Who hates me?*

'You know…people.'

Could rats shrug? *I don't worry so much about what others think about me. It's what I think about myself that's important.*

'Ah, a philosopher rat.'

*What about you?*

'What about me?'

*What do you think about yourself?*

She paused a moment before answering. It was a surprisingly big question for such a small rat. 'I think I'm hard to love.' Her throat thickened around the last word and tears moistened her eyes. She'd never admitted that to anyone before. But it made sense. Her parents practically abandoned her at the first opportunity. Her siblings barely acknowledged her existence. Then again, she didn't make much of an effort with them either.

The rat digested her statement, along with more celery. *Are you really? Or is that just the story you tell yourself?*

Was she really getting into this with a rat? 'Well, health-wise, I'm a mess. I hate the idea of being a burden to anyone. I don't like most people, so I guess that makes it hard for them to like me. I can be snarky and irrational. I'm a liar.' She thought about Krish and how she hadn't trusted him with her secrets, when he was pretty much the most trustworthy person she'd ever met. 'And I'm a coward.'

*Wow. Okay. That's a lot of self-loathing in one go. Now tell me your positive qualities.*

Francesca hugged Hot Willy and examined her toes. She counted each one to make sure they were all there.

*I'm waiting.*

'Just…give me a second. I'm thinking.'

*You shouldn't have to think that hard.*

'Okay. Okay. What about this? I'm generally quite clean.'

*Excuse me?*

'I mean, I take a shower almost every day, so…yeah. I'm clean.' That being said, she remembered the time Krish found her in her office after not sleeping for three days. She hadn't been very clean then.

*Really? That's all you can think of that you like about yourself?*

Krish's words came back to her. 'Well, somebody else said he thought I was strong and stubborn—not sure if that one is a positive —talented...and funny, if you can believe it.'

*And are you?*

Was she?

Francesca attempted to reframe herself with those adjectives. *Strong*: she supposed that she did put up with a lot. She was so used to it by now that it was second nature. *Stubborn*: maybe she'd turn that into a more positive word, like *focused*. Once she got an idea, it was hard to shake—Exhibit A being the entire situation with Krish. But it also meant she was hard-working. It took a lot of focus to stick to her food and exercise regime. *Talented*: actually, yeah. She was good at her job; not great at running a business, but good at her job. She loved observing other people and telling their stories through her lens. In a way, it put a layer of safety between her and real life, just how she liked it. She could be around people—without having to interact with them. *Funny*: well, she was talking to a rat, so...

'I guess I am,' she finally replied. Inside of her, a spark kindled to life.

*Lady, all you need to do is decide to love yourself. The rest will follow. And I'm telling you this as the child of a mother who tried to eat me.*

'Ew. Gross.'

*Listen, I'm late. Gotta get some of this food back to the nest. You know what you gotta do.*

On cue, King Rat turned and disappeared into the wall. Francesca gently closed the cupboard door and shook her head to clear it. What the hell was that? Had she accidentally taken drugs? Was she on some sort of yellow-brick-road-themed trip where wise side characters imparted life lessons? She'd already met Jaiveer the Dancing Scarecrow and the Tin Rat...was the cowardly lion going to knock on her door later and try to sell her overpriced household items while explaining the meaning of life?

She filled her cheeks with air and slowly blew it out. Despite the decidedly trippy nature of the encounter, that rat had given her a lot to think about.

Her stomach grumbled, reminding her that she hadn't eaten any dinner yet. She stood up and went to her fridge.

As she pulled out ingredients from the vegetable bin, she considered the rat's message: *love thyself*. She hated it when pithy, trite sayings that people embroidered on cushions or printed on mugs turned out to be true. How could something so simple be so profound?

But King Rat was right. So much of her mental energy went to telling herself that she was broken and unloveable. If she was ever going to get the happy ending that Jaiveer said she deserved, then her negative self-talk needed to stop.

She snorted as she peeled a carrot. *Easier said than done*. Then again, look what happened when she focussed on making new friends. In one night, she'd already made two (sort of).

As she washed lettuce in a salad spinner, her thoughts returned to Krish and his imminent proposal. Suddenly the breath caught in her throat and she found it hard to inhale. A sob ripped out of her mouth. Sadness and loss rolled through her and she had to lean on the counter to steady herself. Pain that had nothing to do with her uterus erupted in her belly.

All the good times she'd had with Krish scrolled through her head like a slideshow at a funeral. Salty tears fell from her cheek onto the wet lettuce and a quote from *Blade Runner* barged into her head: '*All those moments will be lost in time, like tears in the rain.*'

'Or in the salad spinner,' she hiccuped.

Francesca could see now that she *did* deserve a happy ending, but not at the expense of Krish's. She must take responsibility for her actions and accept the consequences.

She needed to let him go.

## 22

KRISH FINISHED PACKING his suitcase and set it on its feet near the bedroom door. The smell of stir fry and teriyaki wafted through his flat, making his stomach growl.

'Dinner's ready!' Jess called from the kitchen.

Before joining her, he visited the bathroom to throw some water on his face. Since Francesca had firmly slammed the door on them and he'd decided to move ahead with Jess, everything had slotted into place, confirming that he was on the right path. Dinner at his sister's had been surprisingly fun. The four of them had laughed and joked, like they had many times before. Contrary to his fear, it didn't feel weird, and the guilt he'd expected over his kiss with Francesca didn't materialise. In fact, he barely thought about it. Francesca's refusal to tell him the truth about whatever was going on with her and her convenient boyfriends told him he was making the right call.

Perhaps it was a good thing. It allowed him to purge her from his life once and for all.

Ankita didn't know that Krish was planning to propose in Paris, but from the way his sister looked at him with that annoying smirk after he mentioned the upcoming trip, she'd probably figured it out. Nothing got past her.

He was relieved when Francesca wasn't in the office on Monday. Her presence would only have been a distraction, and he had a long To Do list. He'd met with another couple about photographing their wedding, finished retouching the album images for the gangster's daughter, and had reached out to some venues to discuss creating business partnerships.

In addition, he made the most awkward phone call of his life to ask Jess's father for her hand in marriage. Krish wanted to do this right, but her parents lived too far away to ask face-to-face. Her father was one of those dads who was constantly joking, but never funny. Krish almost choked when his future father-in-law quipped, 'You know you're asking the wrong person?' It took Krish a moment to understand his jest.

Anyway, Krish had accomplished a lot in four days.

This felt good. It felt right.

He threw more water on his face and patted the moisture off with a towel. He avoided meeting his own gaze in the mirror.

At dinner, Jess talked excitedly about the antique market she wanted to visit in Paris tomorrow afternoon. She was keen to add to her collection of tacky cookie jars.

He really hated those cookie jars. Some of them gave him the creeps, especially one in particular: a 1950s chef with rosy cheeks, a rotund belly, and a self-satisfied grin. He looked like he had eaten both all the pies and all the children.

Scanning the tasteful, uncluttered decor of his flat, he wondered where they'd put both her teddy bear and her cookie jar collections when she moved in.

Krish shivered.

'You okay?' Jess asked.

'Fine! Just...a chill.'

'Someone must have walked over your grave.'

'Huh?' That sounded ominous.

'That's what my grandma used to say when somebody shivered like that.'

'Oh.'

'Anyway, after the antiques market...' Jess went on to list more things she wanted to do in Paris. It was her first time, and she was understandably excited. He had wanted to go to Morocco, where he'd never been with any previous partners. He had a romantic idea of proposing in the Atlas Mountains, or maybe in a hot air balloon over the desert, but Jess wanted to visit Paris for their anniversary. She didn't like exotic travel as much as he did.

Not that Morocco really qualified as 'exotic' in his book. When he'd first met Jess, she'd never even been outside the UK. Their discussions about holiday destinations involved a lot of compromise, mostly on his part. She vetoed his idea of the Vietnam cycling tour and the Inca Trail expedition. Instead, they went to Bruges and Florence. Great places, but he loved more adventurous destinations. Maybe he could talk her around one day.

Jess said, 'I've heard amazing things about the Tuileries Garden. Have you been?'

Yes. With Francesca.

He recalled sitting by the pond in the garden overlooked by the ornate palace, watching children race their boats on the water. A little girl was having trouble reaching her sailboat with the stick she'd been given, her arms just a tad too short. Krish had helped her retrieve it. The child laughed as he pretended to fall in the water. Wanting to share the moment with Francesca, he turned to smile at her, but she'd disappeared (returning five minutes later with some bottles of water). Three weeks later, Norman happened.

Thinking back to how perfect things had seemed on that holiday, how *promising*, it still shook him to his core that he completely missed that she wasn't happy. For a long time, it made him question his ability to read people—a talent, up until that point, he would have claimed in spades. As far as he was concerned, that trip cemented their new love, boding well for many more trips in the future. They even kept a running list of all the amazing places they'd visit together on his fridge.

How wrong he'd been.

'Yes, it's lovely,' he said to Jess. 'We can go there after the Louvre.'

The Louvre. He and Francesca had laughed their way through that museum, making up stories about what was going on in the paintings. They eschewed the more popular items, avoiding the Mona Lisa in favour of quieter exhibits, feeling like explorers in an Indiana Jones film. They'd discovered intricate artefacts in dark corners: ancient Greek tablets carrying hidden messages, carved urns containing secrets. In the Egyptian room, they made out behind a pillar.

It would be hard to top that experience.

Jess stood to clear the table. 'No,' said Krish. 'You cooked. I'll clean.'

'What did I ever do to deserve you?' She gave him a kiss and went to lounge on the sofa with a glass of wine.

As he filled the sink, he ran through the details of the trip in his head. Tomorrow morning, they'd catch the Eurostar early. He'd bought first-class tickets and booked rooms at the George Cinq. On Saturday night, they'd get on a private boat. As they took a leisurely ride on the Seine, a waiter would serve them a meal cooked by a Michelin-starred chef. They'd finish the journey in front of the Eiffel Tower at dusk. From the bridge, the photographer he'd hired would capture the moment that Krish got down on his knee and proposed. The following day, Krish and Jess would do a two-hour couples shoot with the same photographer in the streets of Paris before catching the train back to London.

He really had thought of everything. Krish wanted to give Jess an unforgettable proposal story, something that would make her teacher friends exclaim with delight. Even if proposing in Paris might be a bit cliché, he was determined to make it the best damned cliché it could be. Only a handful of his friends from Uni were married, and he knew none of them had executed proposals half as romantic as this.

He'd definitely earn all the unicorn stickers.

So why did his stomach ache?

*Must be indigestion.* He let the dirty water out of the sink and went to look for antacids in his bathroom cupboard. There were none.

No problem. He would just run out to the supermarket around the corner and pick some up. 'I'll be back in a minute,' he said to Jess, who was watching *Sex and the City* reruns. 'Do you need anything while I'm out?'

'All good, thanks.'

Out in the warm night air, Krish plunged his hands into his pockets and took a deep breath, raising his shoulders towards his ears. A little of the tension he'd been holding all week dribbled away as he released his shoulders back down and cracked his neck left and right, a habit he'd picked up from Connor.

Actually, Krish could use the walk.

It had been a busy week. He'd filled up every second of his time, leaving no spare moments for second-guessing himself. Since seeing Francesca last Friday, he'd gone out for a run every evening before bed, sometimes late at night. He found that physical exercise helped him have deep, dreamless sleeps—exactly what he needed right now.

He emptied his mind of thought and concentrated on his breathing, taking in the world around him. He noticed the cat in someone's window. The noise of a child crying. Music and conversation from the pub. A siren. The lingering herbal smell of a joint.

Inside the supermarket, he perused the aisles until he found the antacids. Grabbing a box, he turned to go back to the register, but a bright display snagged his eye.

It was the feminine hygiene section. He blinked at the rows of tampons, and his thoughts jumped automatically to Francesca. He wondered if her PMS was better now. Living with that must be horrible, like being a stranger in your own body. When he considered all the things that women had to go through—periods, child-birth, menopause—it made him grateful to be a man.

What was Francesca doing right now? Probably out with friends. Or perhaps she'd be working late. She worked so hard. It made him worry about her, even though, if there was any woman who could take care of herself, it was Francesca.

Another memory of Paris came to him: as they were strolling along the pavement, a Frenchman had squeezed Francesca's bottom while Krish was ahead of her. She turned and punched the sleaze bag in the nuts. As he limped off, an elderly French lady who had seen the whole thing and was wheezing with laughter asked them to join her at her café table and share a bottle of wine.

They'd ended up staying there for hours, chatting with her as she chain smoked cigarette after cigarette. In a deep, throaty voice, she'd said in heavily accented English: 'Remember, if you see some-body walking and smoking in Paris, they aren't true Parisiennes. We always stand still or sit to enjoy our cigarettes. Like civilised people.'

Afterwards, Krish and Francesca had wandered around Montmartre doing a tally of walking versus sitting smokers. A busker sang a song from *Moulin Rouge!*, Francesca's favourite movie, in front of the Sacre Coeur, and they danced together like they were the only two people in the world.

He laughed. It had been one of those impromptu evenings that only ever happened when travelling.

Someone coughed. Krish refocused on the present. A woman was standing nearby, waiting for him to stop gurning at tampons and get out of her way.

He took a step back. 'Um, sorry...'

With nothing else to say, he turned on one foot and raced to the register to pay for his antacids. Outside, he leaned back against a brick wall and tapped his head against the scratchy stone, wishing that it could knock these recurring thoughts of Francesca out of his brain.

But it was no use. Every time he tried to ignore her, her presence grew stronger and brighter. His feelings refused to behave.

What did he love about her, anyway? She could be stroppy and argumentative, bad-tempered, sarcastic and an all-around pain in the arse...but she also cracked him up. Their senses of humour were perfectly in sync. Funny observations that he would have to explain to Jess, Francesca got straight away. And he liked how she used to go out of her way to make him laugh. A few weeks after they started going out, he caught flu over Halloween, so she made him vegetable soup and cooked a hand out of puff pastry to stick in the broth, like a body trying to escape. Since then, he'd secretly believed soup without puff pastry hands was inferior soup. On top of that, she had so much passion. Talented, too. When she smiled, it lit up his heart. And something about her brought out his protective side. He wanted to keep her safe. Make her feel loved and wanted.

And Jess...well, she was easygoing, loyal, and enthusiastic. Sexy, kind and generous. They had fun together. She cared for him.

But Francesca...

*The heart wants what the heart wants.*

He smashed the heels of his hands into his eye sockets and rubbed. How could he propose to one woman when his thoughts were filled with another?

It dawned on Krish that he stood at a crossroads. Life was littered with them—the big ones that would fundamentally change his course. Choosing which university to attend. Choosing to leave the law firm and pursue photography. Choosing to separate from Connor and strike out on his own.

If he had chosen any other path, his life would look completely different right now. He had never been cowed by choosing the harder path in the past, but this one felt different. This time, somebody he loved could get really hurt. Jess was an amazing person. She didn't deserve to have her heart broken.

But she also didn't deserve to have a partner who wasn't 100% focused on her.

He thought about his father and the choices he'd made that resulted in Ankita and Krish: leaving his family in India to study in the UK. Choosing to remain after he graduated. Marrying a white woman despite the disapproval of his parents and society at the time.

How did his father know what to do? The urge to talk to his dad hit Krish strongly, right in his chest, causing it to tighten. *What would Dad say?* He was a man obsessed by science and logic. A man who loved a good plan and seeing it through to fruition. But in this situation, would he counsel his son to follow his heart like he had? Or would he tell Krish to follow his plan? To stay the course?

He could follow through with his proposal to Jess, and they'd probably have an uncomplicated life together. He'd convinced himself that a 'nice' and 'easy' marriage was what he wanted above all else, like his parents. But was that really his dream? He'd always wonder—and always regret—that he hadn't figured out this thing between him and Francesca. He still didn't believe she had a boyfriend. Why was she lying? Whatever happened, he was determined to uncover the answer.

Pressure built in the skin of his hands, blood pooling in his fingers, making them tingle uncomfortably. He made fists, squeezing and releasing a few times to encourage circulation. He slipped his left hand into his pocket, stroking a phantom velvet box containing an antique ring.

He had to make a choice. Jess or Francesca. What should he do?

## 23

FRANCESCA SIPPED her coffee and watched the front door of the office building from the safety of the cafe across the road.

Krish had instructed the whole team for the Blenheim job to arrive at 11AM so they could help pack the equipment into the van before heading straight to the Mehndi Party in Oxfordshire.

Over the weekend, while Krish was still in Paris, Francesca had gone in to water the plants and prep her kit, which she'd left in a pile next to the door, ready to load.

Part of her argued that she had done this while he wasn't there so she could concentrate on making sure she had everything she needed without his distracting presence. But the other, scared part of her knew it was because she didn't want to see him yet, all shiny and newly engaged.

Would he act differently towards her? Colder? More aloof?

At 10:45, a silver minibus pulled up in front of the white stucco building opposite and Krish got out. Her heart pounded at the sight of him. She lifted her large sunglasses to get a better look. Something was different about him, but she couldn't put her finger on what it was. An engaged glow? She wished she could see him more clearly.

Without turning in her direction, he windmilled his arms to get a good stretch and cricked his neck before disappearing through the front door.

A few minutes later, Stella arrived in the company of a ridiculously handsome man and a child. Francesca recognised Connor Knight and Grace. How nice that they came to see her off. The perfect little family.

*No, Francesca.* She gave herself a mental slap. She couldn't keep being angry at people for being happy just because she wasn't. *Love thyself*, she repeated the rat's message.

Krish emerged from the building carrying some of Francesca's kit. He put the items down as Grace toddled towards him and swept her up, as though she weighed nothing. Both of them were laughing. He tilted her body downwards and blew a raspberry on her stomach.

He was so natural with kids, whether they were biologically related to him or not. The way Grace was laughing in his arms was proof of that. Why hadn't she seen that sooner? Why hadn't she trusted him with her secret? Her life could be so different right now.

But it wasn't.

Connor kissed Stella deeply, holding her face between his hands. God, Francesca wanted to be kissed like that. He took Grace, waved, and walked back towards the tube station. Good. Francesca didn't think she could handle meeting *the* Connor Knight right now, on top of everything else.

Krish packed the bags into the van, closed the boot, and disappeared back into the building with Stella.

Popping two co-codamol in her mouth, Francesca washed them down with the last of her lukewarm coffee. Standing, she squared her shoulders. She grabbed the bag of road trip snacks that she'd bought, and left the haven of the cafe, dragging her suitcase behind her across the road. In the lobby, she parked her luggage next to the reception desk and greeted Mick.

'Hey, Francesca.'

'What trash you reading today?'

'*Crime and Punishment.*'

'Another feel-good story, then.' Unzipping her luggage, she pulled out a book. 'I brought something for you. I thought you might like to read one of the most important feminist works of the 20<sup>th</sup> century.' She handed him her worn copy of *Bridget Jones's Diary*. 'Make sure you return it. I have notes in the margin.'

'Thanks,' he said, taking it from her with an appreciative smile. 'I will.'

*Okay, I can't avoid seeing Krish any longer.* She stowed her bags next to the reception desk and pushed the lift call button. Too fast, it came. She stepped inside, her apprehension growing with every movement.

*Here goes nothing.*


UPSTAIRS, THE OFFICE DOOR WAS WEDGED OPEN. FRANCESCA STOPPED just outside for a moment, to indulge in a few deep breaths. She was glad Stella was there—Francesca didn't think she could handle being alone with newly-engaged Krish just yet.

His deep, resonant voice floated through the door, and her ears devoured every word: 'Let's bring those bags to the van first.' He could make anything sound sexy.

Stella replied with excitement, 'I refuse to take anything until you tell me how the proposal went!'

Francesca's feet moved before she'd even sent the command. She'd be damned if she was going to listen to this story. She stepped into the room.

Krish and Stella both startled, like they'd been caught planning a murder. Francesca didn't miss the look that passed between them: *We'll talk about this later.*

Her cramps chose that moment to ignite, the co-codamol yet to work its magic. Her facial muscles tightened with the effort it took to hide the ache. Thank goodness for big sunglasses. Right now they were keeping all of Francesca's secrets: the puffy residue of a week full of tears, the pain, her feelings for Krish.

'You shaved,' she said, glad he couldn't see the joy in her eyes. *Alleluia, the hair was gone.*

He rubbed his newly shorn jawline. 'Needed a change.'

'I like it better.' Seeing him without his beard...It did things to her, and she couldn't help but gawk. The Krish of five years ago had reappeared. His dimples seemed to be waving at her, freed from their hairy prison. She wondered why he'd done it.

His own gaze flicked up and down her body and she hoped he approved of her choice of clothing: colourful green trousers and a matching sleeveless top, embroidered with bright pink flowers and tiny mirrors, Indian-inspired. She had made a real effort to wear something appropriate for this specific wedding.

Stella cleared her throat.

Krish shook his head as though snapping himself out of a spell. 'Apologies. This is Francesca—'

'Actually, we've already met,' Stella said. 'I popped by last Thursday. Francesca was kind enough to entertain me while Grace slept.'

If it didn't make her so sad, Francesca might have laughed at his momentary look of panic. She could practically hear him wondering if Stella had spilled the beans about the proposal, not that Francesca was going to bring it up. In any case, they couldn't stand there all day awkwardly staring at each other. 'Shall we get this show on the road?' Francesca said.

As they loaded up with bags, she contemplated how she should act towards him. Should she pretend everything was fine between them? Amicable? She reminded herself that a) he was engaged to Jess, b) they had a huge wedding job to do, and c) the last time she'd seen him, she pretty much booted him out of her life.

*Just be natural,* said her inner Brooklyn-accented rat.

Easier said than done when she found herself pressed up against him in the lift. Stella had insisted on taking the stairs while Krish and Francesca rode down with the kit. She wondered if Stella had done it on purpose, a misguided attempt to give them a chance to talk.

Krish cleared his throat. 'Good weekend?'

'Yup.' She wasn't going to volley the question back. She didn't want to know. It still hurt that he had taken Jess to Paris, which Francesca very much considered *their* city. For a moment, she flipped through proposal locations again, but then stopped herself. Dwelling on it wasn't very self-loving and did not serve her mental health. King Rat would be proud.

Instead, she concentrated on the metallic lift wall, where some industrial wordsmith had scratched *I love balls*. But it was hard to concentrate on anything when Krish smelled so damned good. Like citrus and spice. His t-shirt left his arms bare, the sleeves struggling to wrap themselves around his ample muscles. Behind her sunglasses, her eyes rolled back in her head as she inhaled deeply. She noted that her mouth was tantalisingly close to his bicep, and the sudden urge to lick him came upon her. She clamped her teeth shut.

*Ding.*

The lift door opened, breaking through the sex show playing in her mind.

'After you,' he said, shifting so she could exit first. Ever the gentleman.

Whatever the female equivalent of ball ache was, she had that.

As they left the building, the muggy air hit her in the face, making her sunglasses slip down her nose. That was the cost of a beautiful summer wedding with blue skies: hideous heat. At least the van would have air conditioning.

She saw a small East Asian boy waiting next to the van with a heavy kit bag almost half his size. He must be her drone operator. He looked like he was heading off to his first day of high school in an American film: new backpack looped over both shoulders and a light blue dress shirt, sharply ironed and tucked into spotless tan trousers. His trainers glowed white. Was this work experience or a job? She pondered whether his parents had dropped him off. 'David Yun?' she asked.

'That's me!' He picked up his bag. 'Do you mind if we put her on top? Lucy can be a bit delicate.'

'Lucy?' Francesca said, worried that he'd also packed a small animal.

'My drone.'

Krish coughed next to her, and she knew he was disguising his laughter. 'Sure, David,' he said. 'I'm Krish.'

The drone operator shook Krish's hand with the exuberant zeal of a puppy going to a butt-sniffing party. Up close, his glasses were so thick that, for a second, she knew what bugs felt like under a microscope.

Francesca, Stella, and David made two more trips upstairs for the bags while Krish packed everything into the van like a master Tetris player. Finished, he slammed the hatch and looked at his watch. 'Any idea where your other camera man is?' he asked, addressing Francesca.

'I told him 11AM sharp.' She checked her watch. It was already twenty past. *Shit.* What if Wally let her down? Krish would think she was such an amateur.

'G'day! Sorry I'm late. Tube troubles.'

They all turned towards a young man sporting a pink mohawk, black skinny jeans, and a white t-shirt. The word DEATH was tattooed down the middle of his neck. He dropped his kit on the ground and adjusted the rucksack on his shoulder.

'Wally?' said Francesca. When she'd worked with him years ago, he'd been fresh from Oz, with a tanned, muscular build and a mop of sun-bleached blond hair. London had changed him.

'You can call me Wazza, if you want,' he said.

She didn't want. She glanced at Krish, worried how he'd react to the fact that she had hired a punk covered in satanic tattoos to work a traditional Indian wedding. 'Hey, Wazza. I'm Krish. Do you want to keep your bag or put it in the boot?'

He seemed unperturbed. David, on the other hand, was staring at their new colleague like an alien had just landed and asked for directions to parliament.

'Aw, I'll hold onto it. Cheers, mate.'

Everyone climbed into the van: Wally at the back, Stella and David in the middle, and Francesca riding at the front with Krish, who settled himself into the driver seat, adjusting the mirrors. She turned on the radio and, pitching her voice low so no one but Krish could hear, said, 'Sorry, I didn't know about...' She tilted her head towards Wally.

'Only thing I care about is whether he can do the job. Can he?'

She nodded and hoped she was telling the truth.

'Good. Well then. No problem.' He paused and looked her square in the eyes. 'I've come to be a big believer in the idea that everything happens for a reason.'

They held eye contact, and she wanted so badly to ask him what he meant by that. Was he referring to her coming back into his life? Or his getting engaged to Jess? Or the way Netflix cancelled seasons prematurely?

*What?* Her heart screamed for the answer.

Instead, she broke the trance and dropped her gaze to the radio.

'Francesca?' he said, pulling her attention back to him.

'Yeah?'

Leaning towards her, Krish said, 'Why do I feel like I've formed some sort of crazy heist team, like in *Oceans Eleven*?'

She offered half a smile. 'Well, the good news is...that makes you George Clooney.'

'And who does that make you?' He shifted the van into drive and put on the indicator.

'I'm the smart one,' she said with a wink.

'The Elliott Gould character?'

Gould played the Jewish ex-casino owner who spoke with the same accent as King Rat. 'Oh, yeah. I'm definitely Elliott Gould.'

They laughed. It felt good to let herself laugh with him.

. . .

TWO HOURS LATER, THEY ARRIVED AT ISHANI'S PARENTS' HOUSE IN Oxfordshire.

Stella had worked at some amazing family estates in her days photographing with Connor, but this one rivalled them all in opulence. 'What do they do for a living?' she asked as the van emerged from the cypress-lined drive and they found themselves in front of a wonder of modern architecture, all clean white concrete and sleek glass. It screamed Bond Criminal.

'They're the biggest importer of Indian food in the UK,' Krish said.

*That's a lot of poppadoms*, thought Stella.

They parked at the edge of the large, circular forecourt, between the vehicles of the florist and caterer. The event wouldn't start until later that evening, but according to the schedule, the couple wanted to do a series of shoots on the grounds in various outfits before the guests arrived. Standard stuff.

Francesca announced that she was going to find a toilet and leapt out of the van. Krish unloaded the boot's contents onto the mani- cured grass and then climbed into the boot to use it as a changing room. He emerged a few minutes later in a white button-down shirt and grey trousers. The rest of them found their bags and headed to the shade of a nearby oak, out of the sun's brutal rays.

'I can carry that for you,' offered Wally.

'Thanks.' Stella let him pick up her heavy roller bag. They'd spoken for part of the journey about the Australian towns she'd visited on her trip with Connor, and they trotted out that conversa- tion that non-Australians always had with Australians about how all the nature there is designed to kill people. Wally said that's why he'd moved to the UK, because he was afraid of snakes.

The light-hearted chat had helped to calm her nerves. But now, it was show time, and her stomach feathered with anxiety. Would she remember how to work a wedding?

'You can do this,' Stella muttered to herself as she took out her camera and slung the strap around her neck. It felt like an old friend in her hands. She relaxed a little.

Her phone buzzed and she smiled. It was probably Connor calling to wish her good luck. She checked the screen and was surprised to see not her husband's name, but Claudia's.

'Oh, hey! All okay?' Stella asked.

'Quick question. Can Grace eat peanut butter?' Claudia said in a raised voice, vying with the sounds of screaming children in the background.

'Yes, but…why?' Grace was supposed to be having some daddy/daughter time.

Claudia phewed with relief. 'Thank fuck for that. Because she's already had some.'

Stella turned away from the others and tried to keep her voice calm. 'Why is she even there?'

'Connor asked if he could leave Grace with us for the afternoon. Something about interviews? It's no problem. The twins love her.'

Annoyance bubbled up, temporarily curbing Stella's anxiety about the wedding. 'Thanks, Clauds. I appreciate your checking. What time is he picking her up, out of interest?'

'Around eight or so?'

That was well past Grace's bedtime. Connor would mess up Stella's new sleep schedule. After the dysregulation of their trip, she was trying to get her daughter into bed by six o'clock every night after a bath and stories. Routine. All the baby books said that it was important at this age. 'I've got to go, Clauds. Tell Grace I love her.' Stella hung up and let out an exasperated sigh.

'What's wrong?' asked Krish, who was formatting his cards nearby.

'Nothing. Connor is supposed to be watching Grace. We even went over all the things he could do with her while I was away.' What a waste of an hour. Had he ever planned on spending any time with his daughter?

'And...?'

Her voice rose despite trying to control it, and her Italian hands flailed angrily. 'And he's just dumped her at Claudia's so he can go to his studio to interview replacements for you.'

'Maybe you just got your wires crossed.'

It hurt that Krish was making excuses for Connor. At least she knew where his loyalties lay. 'Yeah, well that seems to be the status quo these days.'

Krish touched her arm. 'Everything okay?'

She rubbed at her temples. It had been unfair thinking ill of Krish. 'Oh, yeah. It's nothing. We just...seem to be having a few hiccups with settling back into home life, that's all.'

He sounded sad when he said, 'Why do relationships have to be so hard?'

She huffed a laugh. 'Don't worry, I'm sure Jess will be more of a team player than Connor.'

Krish paused a moment, checking behind him before saying in a low voice: 'I didn't propose.'

'Shit! Krish! No! What happened?' Her own problems suddenly seemed less important.

'I broke up with her. I feel absolutely terrible about it—and guilty as hell. She went off to Paris alone instead. Something about wanting to get closure.' Stella reached out and grabbed his hand. 'I just...' His eyes were following something past her shoulder. Stella glanced back and saw it was Francesca returning from the toilets. 'I just realised that she wasn't who I wanted to spend my life with.'

So her hunch had been right! There *was* something going on between Francesca and Krish. And judging from how she reacted when Stella mentioned the Paris Proposal, Francesca had feelings for him, too. Stella was dying to tell him about what happened when she'd visited the office, but she promised Francesca she wouldn't say anything. They'd have to sort this one out all on their own. 'Well, I hope it all works out for you,' she said, rubbing his arm.

Krish glanced down at his watch. 'Speaking of matrimonial bliss, the bride will be expecting you and Francesca soon.'

Her stomach flipped. This was it. Just like riding a bike, right?

*Tits and teeth*, she said to herself, repeating her old mantra from her competitive dancing days as she made her way towards the house, trying not to dwell on her husband's deception.

## 24

FRANCESCA AND STELLA started with the bride while Krish and Wally went in search of the groom. He would arrive by helicopter in the fields out back. *Like the mega-wanker he is,* thought Francesca.

Inside the modern marvel of a house, she admired the amount of time and effort that must have gone into hanging that many flowers. Ropes of jasmine and multi-coloured marigolds covered the walls, dangled from the chandelier, ran along the bannisters. It smelled heavenly. They must have cost a fortunate and this wasn't even the main event.

Stella and Francesca carefully made their way up the glass stair-case in search of the bride, each of them trying to lug their heavy kit without chipping the stairs. Having glass stairs seemed about as practical as wearing a glass slipper.

After peeking into several empty guest rooms, they eventually found Ishani in a crisp, clean bedroom with floor-to-ceiling windows overlooking the back garden. Inside her head, Francesca did a mini fist pump. The natural light in this room was soft, plenti-ful, and perfect.

Francesca greeted Ishani and introduced Stella.

Scanning Stella up and down, Ishani demanded, 'Where's Krish?'

'Um…' said Stella. Francesca was surprised to see Stella falter at Ishani's harsh tone, struggling for words.

'I don't mean to be difficult, but our contract is with Krish,' the bride said, every inch the lawyer. 'Where is *he*?'

Stella's shoulders dipped, and her smile faltered. Were those tears? When she'd stopped by the office the week before, she confessed she was nervous because she hadn't shot a wedding in a year and a half. And on her first job back, she got a bridezilla. Poor woman.

Unused to being in a management position, it occurred to Francesca that she was the senior supplier under Krish. On one hand, she had to keep the client happy, especially if Krish wanted the Mumbai wedding, too. On the other hand, she couldn't let Ishani destroy Stella's confidence. A strange fizzle started in her stomach which felt oddly like…responsibility.

If only diplomacy were her forte. She was not known for her honeyed words and delicate negotiations. But for Krish, she could try.

'Don't you know who this bloody well is?' said Francesca, matching Ishani's tone and willing her face into a mask of calm even as her uterus twisted. The co-codamol chose exactly that moment to wear off.

Ishani's eyebrows shot into the air, and Francesca continued, 'Stella Price-Knight has photographed *everybody* who's *anybody*, and frankly you're lucky she was available. She's one of the best. THE BEST.' Stella looked embarrassed and gratified by the praise. 'You gave us a long list of shots to take that would be *physically impossible* for one photographer to do on his own. So, in order to fulfil *your requirements*, Krish has put together an amazing team. You're welcome.'

The room was silent for a moment as the words settled. Even the make-up and hair artists hovering in the corner stopped moving. All eyes were on the bride, awaiting her reaction.

'Stella Price-Knight! Of course,' Ishani said in a complete about-face, as though she'd just been talking about Stella's work in *Vogue* with her mates last weekend. 'I hope I didn't offend you.'

'No, not at all,' said Stella, standing tall again. She threw a thankful smile at Francesca and launched into a discussion with Ishani about her ideas and possible locations.

Francesca smiled, delighted with her burst of diplomatic prowess. Then her smile faltered. She wondered how she'd explain Wally.

Maybe they wouldn't notice.

After that, things went smoothly. Stella appeared to regain her confidence, coaching Ishani into pose after pose and finding just the right light. Francesca and Stella worked well together, and she didn't try to hog the bride like a lot of other photographers. She made sure to give Francesca time to film what she needed, too.

To be fair, there were harder jobs than getting good photos of Ishani.

She practically glowed in her lehenga. The sleeveless top shimmered with champagne crystals and left her toned midriff bare. Her floor-length skirt was covered in soft rose-coloured feathers that floated as she walked. Francesca wondered how many Fraggles had been scalped to make that skirt. Whatever the answer, it was worth it.

Ishani's henna had already been applied a couple days before to give the colours time to fully bloom. The brown lines laced around the bride's forearms, gossamer strokes ending in a cuff of flowers just below her elbow. In the middle of her right palm, the henna artist had drawn a detail-perfect picture of the bride and groom and, on the left, an exact likeness of Fufu, the dog...

...who was currently having her anal glands expressed by a groomer in the bathroom. Francesca tried to ignore the fishy smell as they finished up with the bride.

'Paramjeet incoming. Over,' Krish said through her earpiece, helicopter blades whirring in the background. An involuntary shiver rolled through her as his voice caressed the hairs in her inner ear. He sounded so close, like he was standing next to her and whispering.

These headpieces were another first for Francesca. Due to the size of the wedding and the team, Krish had bought walkie talkie sets for everyone to keep them in close contact. Each person had a speaker nestled in their ear, a microphone clipped on the necklines of their top, and a receptor unit weighing down the waistline of their trousers. Having the earpiece in place took some getting used to, but now she didn't really notice it.

Depressing the talk button on the mic, Francesca replied like she had been trucking all her life. 'Ten-four. On our way with the bride. Over.'

FIVE HOURS AND FOUR BRIDAL OUTFIT CHANGES LATER, KRISH CHECKED his watch. Guests would be arriving soon—only 150 or so family members and close friends of the bride and groom.

The pair were hard work; one of those extremely gorgeous couples who were so insecure they questioned every creative direction Krish made. If he asked the bride to look left because that was the direction of the light, she'd insist that right showed her better side. If he asked the groom to stand with a slightly wider stance to even out the height difference, he would refuse because he didn't want to look short.

Despite their interference, he'd managed to take some amazing shots. Portfolio-worthy shots. Even the bride and groomzilla should be happy with the results.

The team took a quick dinner break while the bride and groom changed. Again. They sat together on the veranda next to the pool, I & P spelled out on the surface of the water in pink and white lotuses. It was almost 7PM, so most of the day's heat had now gone. Still, it had been a hot one. Tomorrow would be even hotter.

Krish checked in with each of the team to make sure they had everything they needed. Stella was sitting in one of those hanging egg chairs, checking her messages with a scowl on her face. 'All okay?' he asked.

'Yeah. Great,' she said with a flat voice. He assumed she was still angry at Connor.

'I'm fine,' David said between sneezes. Unfortunately, the house was decorated with strings of flowers everywhere, and David had an allergic reaction. Probably the jasmine. His nose streamed, and his eyes had gone puffy and red. The bride's mother had given him an anti-histamine, but it didn't seem to be helping that much. Krish clapped him on the back. 'Try to stay outside the house for the rest of the night.'

David nodded.

'Where's Wally?' Krish said.

'Personally, I'd look for his little red hat first,' said Francesca, who was sitting on a stone bench and finishing up a plate of vegetarian curry.

'Ha ha,' said Krish, cracking a wide smile. 'No really?'

'He went to the toilet.'

Krish took a seat next to her. 'How's the footage looking?' He let his knee fall towards her so that it brushed her leg. She didn't move away. Was that a good sign? Or was she just too tired to bother? Between the heat and the constant challenges from the couple, five hours seemed like twenty.

'Great, actually. The footage with those zebras...'

'I know. Crazy.' Ishani's father kept a herd, and they'd done some close-up shots with one of the tamer zebras.

'You've got to see this one clip.' She put down her paper plate and picked up her camera from the bench next to her. Krish leaned towards her to get a better view. The fact that it brought his upper body into contact with her and he could smell her sweet shampoo was just an added bonus. He could hear her breathe. She always breathed a little heavier when she was concentrating. And when they used to make love, she concentrated *a lot*. Krish fought the urge to nuzzle her hair with his nose.

Completely unaware of his jangled emotions, she scrolled through the clips on her memory card and hit play on one where the zebra butted his head against Paramjeet's bottom, making him step into a pile of soft dung.

They both laughed, indulging in some mutual schadenfreude.

Francesca played it again. 'It probably won't make it into the final f—'

'Goldie?! What are you doing here?'

A voice cut through their conversation, and Krish looked up to see a tall man with a chiselled jaw and short, gelled hair. He wore a loose turquoise kurta pyjama edged in gold, paired with tan trousers and matching slippers.

She practically threw her camera into Krish's lap and ran over to the man, launching herself into his arms so her feet dangled off the ground. Francesca? Hugging voluntarily? Krish sat up straighter.

'Jaiveer!' she cried out happily. 'What are *you* doing here?'

Jaiveer? As in the mystery *boy*friend, Jaiveer? A sour ball formed in Krish's gut.

'I choreographed the dances for the Sangeet and for tomorrow, of course,' he said, returning the hug and adding in a kiss on her cheek.

'I'm filming the wedding!' she said. Jaiveer dropped her to the ground and they both jumped up and down with excitement.

*Seriously*, Krish wondered. *What had happened to Francesca?* He had never seen her like this with anyone else: playful, fun, and silly. Something inside of him ripped, knowing that another man had brought this out in her. Krish wanted to be the one to light her up.

Stepping back, she ran her eyes up and down Jaiveer's body in a way that made Krish clench his jaw. 'I didn't realise you had clothes that weren't black.' She giggled. Francesca actually *giggled*.

*Ha. Ha. Bloody ha*, thought Krish. Personally, he wouldn't trust a man who didn't have some colour in his wardrobe.

'This is Krish,' she said, proffering her hand in his direction. He caught the pointed look that passed between them. So, she'd told Jaiveer about him. Did she mention the kiss? Or just that he was her ex? He suddenly wanted to know, quite badly.

'Nice to meet you.' Jaiveer held out his hand, and Krish shook it.

Annoyingly, it was a good handshake. If it had been too weak or too hard, at least he could have inferred something from it. But this was the handshake of someone who wasn't trying to prove anything and didn't feel threatened. At all.

To Francesca, Jaiveer said, 'Do you know where Paramjeet is?'

'Upstairs, trying to solve world hunger and figure out the plastic crisis.'

'Sounds like him.' They shared a chuckle. 'I'll see you later.' He kissed her on the cheek again and trotted into the house. Krish gritted his teeth.

'What?' said Francesca when she caught Krish's eyes on her.

He shrugged, struggling to look nonchalant while his insides raged. 'Nothing. He seems nice.'

'Yeah, he's great. And such a talented choreographer. He won a Fanfare award, you know.'

*He won a Fanfare award*, Krish repeated in a childish voice in his head, knowing it was beneath him and doing it anyway. He narrowed his eyes. So, Francesca hadn't made up Jaiveer. He was a living, breathing person. She *seemed* comfortable in his company, and he *seemed* like a nice guy.

That being said, something didn't add up.

If they were dating, why didn't they know that they would both be here today? Surely they would have talked about it. And why did he only kiss her on the cheek? Surely, if they were together, they would have kissed on the mouth.

The ex-lawyer in him knew what to do.

'How did you two meet?' he asked.

'He teaches a Bollywood dance class downstairs from my flat,' she said as she attached her camera to a handheld steady-cam rig.

Krish didn't want to think about Jaiveer being in her flat. 'How long have you been dating?'

'Um…about a month.'

Ah, hesitation. Most couples in the throes of early love would know exactly how long they'd been together, down to the hour. 'Where is he from?'

'India.'

'What city?'

'Mumbai?'

Her voice went up at the end, like she wasn't 100% sure. Interesting. 'What film did he win the Fanfare award for?' If there was one thing he knew about Francesca, it was that she hated Bollywood films.

'*Panje ka Nyaay.*'

Okay, he was a little taken aback by her perfect pronunciation and, he had to admit, a tiny bit impressed. That was a great film. And that dance scene with the dogs…a modern classic.

'Why the third degree?' She stopped prepping her kit and glared at him.

'I was just curious.' He crossed his arms.

At that moment, a loud grunt came in over their headsets, followed by a kerplunk and a splash. Stella, David, Krish, and Francesca all touched their ears at the same time.

'What the fuck was that?' asked Francesca.

Stella, her face scrunched up in disgust, said, 'It sounded like…'

'Pooping!' said David with juvenile delight, followed by a sneeze.

Krish put two and two together. He touched the microphone on his shirt collar, pressing the button to broadcast his voice to the whole team. 'Wally? I think your mic is on. Over.'

A moment of silence and then, 'Bugger! Sorry, mate. The button on my thingy gets stuck sometimes. Guess you all got an earful. Over.'

Great, a faulty headset. That was annoying, especially as Krish had paid a lot of money for them.

From the foyer of the house came the salutations of guests arriving. Krish depressed the button on his mic again. 'Don't worry, Wally, we'll fix it later. Just…hurry up. Guests are on site. Over.'

Another plop sounded through the headset. 'Be there shortly, mate. Over,' he said with a strained voice.

Krish picked up his camera from the outdoor dining table and looped the strap around his neck. He would follow up with Francesca about Jaiveer later. As he fiddled with his settings, he prayed to whomever was listening that nothing else at this wedding went to shit.

Francesca quickly realised that she loved Indian weddings almost as much as she loathed traditional English ones.

Since the guests arrived, it had been a whirlwind of colour and sound and scent. Men and women alike were dressed brightly, with lehengas and sarees in every shade of the rainbow. And the delicious smells...the sweet perfume of the hanging flowers mingled with aromatic cumin, frying onions, and zesty garlic; the buffet set up in the garden immediately grew a queue.

The sensual, off-beat percussion of Bhangra music electrified the air. Something about that rhythm made Francesca want to move her feet, more so than the twee pop songs she heard on the radio. She filmed the DJ mixing sounds at his desk near the pool. Beyond him, past where the patio ended, a massive dance floor had been laid, starry lights twinkling across its whole surface. Gently glowing paper lanterns hung from trees surrounding it, and on the far side, there was a low, covered stage with strings of pink and blue flowers hanging down to frame an ornate two-person sofa. Behind the sofa, a bright yellow neon sign proclaimed 'Paramjeet & Ishani'.

Inside the house, a room had been set aside for the henna. The bride's parents had flown in the top mehndi artists from around the world to draw intricate motifs on the guests' hands. When one of the grannies noticed Francesca admiring her designs, the woman explained that the henna stood for good health and prosperity in marriage. Francesca wished she could get it done, too, but the paste took too long to dry.

When the Sangeet started, Francesca fell in love once and for all. If she never worked a traditional English wedding again, it would be too soon. She had seen Sangeet parties in films, but the reality eclipsed those. A Sangeet was like a big dance off between families, a joyous celebration full of music and movement. It felt like being on the set of a Bollywood production with the colourful outfits, the choreographed dancing, and the lavish setting.

First Paramjeet and the younger men from his family took to the floor, including Jaiveer. They performed a group dance, all wearing the groom's signature turquoise and gold. Their movements were exact and well-rehearsed and full of energy. At the end, cold fireworks spurted off the stage behind them. Not to be outdone, Ishani and the ladies, draped in pinks and yellows, pushed the men out of the way for their dance—more feminine and graceful than the men's, but with the same non-stop energy. So. Much. Jumping.

Jaiveer must have rehearsed them all for months to synchronise them so perfectly. The men and women combined for a final show-stopping dance where confetti canons spurted pink and blue paper into the air. Afterwards, the bride and groom sank into their loveseat on the stage and watched performances by the children and a dance-off between members of both their families. The competition was intense, culminating in a final showdown between a cousin from each side. The bride's cousin incorporated a lot of flipping into his. He won in the end, much to the vexation of Paramjeet, who carried on like he'd just lost the FIFA World Cup in a shoot out.

The Bhangra music continued to pump loudly from the speakers: women's high-pitched voices and drum beats that made Francesca's feet itch. The dance floor had opened up to all and overflowed with young and old alike. She recognised at least four famous Bollywood actors among the crowd.

For a beat, she wondered if Krish and Jess would have a wedding like this, full of celebration and joy. Jess would fill out a bridal lehenga well with her svelte goddess body and Francesca didn't even want to imagine how handsome Krish would look. She squeezed her eyes shut and shook her head to dispel the image. Thinking like that would only make her sad and, right now, she wanted to be happy.

Normally, Francesca would film dances from the outskirts, never daring the fray of moving bodies. She didn't want to risk being felt up by Uncle Bob or a horny groomsman either. Also, there was something about dancing in front of others that made her feel exposed.

But at this wedding, the urge to sink into the melee and get some messy, energetic footage overtook her. Maybe it was because of her dance lessons. Maybe the music just made her feel jolly. Whatever it was, she decided to give in to the urge.

Slapping a 50mm lens on her camera, she waded in, hoovering up handheld video of arms in the air, hips gyrating, and bodies bouncing. Her own hips couldn't help but sway to the music.

'Having fun?' shouted Jaiveer next to her.

'This is the best wedding I've ever been to,' she said honestly.

He took her hand, and she let her camera drop around her neck, steadying it with her other hand so it didn't bounce around. They danced next to each other for a few minutes, and she used some of the moves she'd learnt in his class.

'Glad to know you were paying attention.' He smiled. 'Wait until you see the dance tomorrow. I've got fifty professionals taking part.'

She looked up with a huge grin on her face and saw Krish standing on the stage, shooting down towards the rippling horde. His camera concealed his features, but she knew his eye was on her. In a moment of mischief, she turned her back towards Jaiveer and, keeping contact between them, she wiggled her body down to the floor and back up again. That would teach Krish to spy on her.

After a few more minutes, she excused herself. 'I'm still on the clock. See you later.' She threaded her way off the dance floor and found her kit bag to change to a wider lens.

Without warning, a heaviness seeped into her limbs, and her energy dipped, making her head spin. She grabbed the back of a nearby chair to steady herself while the feeling passed. This was another of her many symptoms, exacerbated by the fact that she'd been on her feet for almost ten hours.

She checked the time. Their photography and video service ended soon, and they could head to the B&B to pass out. It would be an early start tomorrow; they were expected at Blenheim by 8AM.

As though she'd sent up a Bat Signal, Krish appeared next to her, ever the knight.

'All okay?' he asked.

'You don't need to check up on me.' She snatched her hand from the chair and stood up straight.

'I'm not,' he said.

She gave him a look.

'Okay, I was. You look tired.'

'Gee, thanks.'

'If it's any consolation, I'm exhausted, too.'

Before she could reply, a fit, middle-aged woman with strong eyebrows, kohled eyes, and a decadently jewelled yellow lehenga sidled up to Krish and asked, without introducing herself, 'Are you married?'

'No?' said Krish with uncertainty. He threw a confused glance at Francesca.

'Wonderful. My name's Divya Verma, India's busiest matchmaker.' She handed over an embossed card with lots of fancy red writing on it.

'Oh?' His whole demeanour changed, his head tilting attentively to the side as though he was all ears. Francesca did not like where this was going.

Divya continued in a strong accent, 'I've had my eye on you this whole night. I think you'd be perfect for one of my clients—a beautiful Gujarati girl, an artist. Her career is up and up. I have a hunch that you'd be a good match. And I am never wrong.'

Francesca studied Krish. He seemed to be considering it! What was he doing? He was already taken, much to her despair. And if she couldn't have him, then neither could this woman and her beautiful *gujju* girl.

'He's engaged,' jumped in Francesca, taking the card out of Krish's hands, ripping it in two, and dropping it to the ground.

'Oh,' the woman said with both surprise and disappointment. 'Well, if it doesn't work out, let me know. I could have you paired off like that.' She snapped her fingers, turned and walked away. Krish groaned.

'What did you do that for?' He bent over and collected the card pieces off the grass.

'Because you're taken! Remember Jess?'

He flinched. Curious. 'Divya Verma is the biggest matchmaker in India! She could single-handedly fill up my bookings for next year.'

'Yeah, well...' The conviction she'd had a moment before fled. She was too tired to fight. 'Sorry.'

'And I'm not, by the way.'

'Not what?'

'Not engaged.'

Nearby, confetti canons fired and multi-coloured tissue paper floated down around them, getting stuck in his hair.

Surely the noise of the canon had obscured what he said. Or her ears weren't working. One of them was blocked up by the walkie talkie speaker, so she must have heard wrong. 'Sorry, what?' A piece of tissue paper attached itself to her lips and she flicked it away.

'I'm not engaged,' he repeated with a tinge of sadness. His umber brown eyes fastened on hers and held tight. She couldn't have looked away if she wanted to, especially because of the pain. *His* pain. His eyes swam with it.

Poor Krish. Did Jess say no?

Or did he decide not to ask? Did he go to Paris at all? Did they break up?

If they'd broken up, did that mean he *wasn't* taken?

She was too afraid to ask. Whatever the answer, he was obviously upset about it. Now was not the time to launch into a cross examination.

The voice of a wise rat cut through the noise: *Just ask him, for chrissake!*

Francesca gulped and gathered her courage. 'Are you...are you still together?'

Her whole body froze with fear, as though she'd woken up from a nightmare but couldn't move, convinced that robe on her door was actually an axe murderer. What he said next could change everything.

'No.'

She exhaled, not realising she'd been holding her breath. The pain in his eyes morphed into something else. A question. She wasn't ready to answer it. 'Well, I'm sorry to hear—'

'May day! May day!' came Stella's voice over the headset, like she was in a plane about to crash.

In a blink, the moment was lost. Krish touched the button on his collar. 'Stella, what's wrong? Over.'

'It's Wally,' she said. 'He's been in a fight and pushed one of the groom's cousins into the pool.'

## 25

NOBODY SPOKE on the half-hour journey to the bed and breakfast.

After the constant craziness of the Mehndi night and the Sangeet, Stella appreciated the silence to decompress. She had forgotten how frenetic weddings could be. The non-stop concentration, always looking for an interesting angle, the endless movement, all on less sustenance than she needed because she was too busy to eat properly. It was like running a marathon after consuming a chocolate bar.

That being said, it had proven a welcome distraction from her anger towards Connor.

When she'd texted him to ask why Grace was at Claudia's, he wrote back (one hour later): **Work emergency. Don't worry Grace happy.**

She texted back, saying she knew he was doing the interviews that she thought he'd cancelled, but he didn't reply.

Aside from his deception, the thing that angered her most was that she'd spent ages putting together a list of daddy-daughter activity ideas for Connor and Grace, trying to make it easy for him. Little did she know that he had no intention of using it. Had he just been humouring her? Wasting her time?

Checking her messages, she noted that he still hadn't replied to the text she'd sent three hours ago, asking if he would be with Grace tomorrow.

Behind her, David sneezed.

Misery was written on his bespectacled face in red splotches and snot. He had soldiered on regardless, never complaining for a moment. What a trooper.

And then there was Wally. Poor Wally. He'd had a truly hard day. It must be so disheartening being judged because of his appearance, especially when, in her opinion, Wally was such a nice guy. At every opportunity, he'd offered to carry her bags, and he was constantly refilling the whole team's water bottles to make sure they stayed hydrated.

One of the groom's cousins had decided as soon as he arrived that he disliked Wally. Stella could see it in the man's eyes whenever he caught sight of Wally's pink mohawk: a curl of the lip, a darkening of the eyes, the stroking of a fist. As a photographer, she caught a lot of subtext while watching people through her lens. That cousin was trouble.

So when he pushed Wally, the third time, Wally finally pushed back. The cousin flew into the pool, ruining the beautiful I & P lotus flower design.

Thankfully, enough people had seen the fight to know that Wally had not started it. Stella got the impression that this particular cousin was known for being an arsehole. After he was fished out of the pool, a bevy of rotund aunties surrounded him, berating him for being a *gadha*, whatever that meant.

Their van pulled up outside the bed and breakfast, ablaze with welcoming light despite the late hour. Everyone collected their bags and piled into the nondescript pebble-dashed house, where the host showed them each to their rooms: Stella and Francesca were next to each other; Krish was down the hall; David and Wally were upstairs.

Nobody spoke, too exhausted to form words. They had to do it all over again tomorrow.

Stella was asleep before her head hit the pillow.

. . .

KRISH DROVE THE VAN UP THE LONG DRIVEWAY TO BLENHEIM PALACE. In the rearview mirror, he flicked his eyes towards Francesca in the passenger seat. She was still staring out the window, as she had done since they left the B&B.

Since confessing to her that he wasn't engaged, he had tried to speak with her alone. But she seemed to have other plans. Last night at the B&B, she'd run into her room and closed the door with a firm slam. That morning, she came out for breakfast last and left first.

He had hoped her reaction would be different.

What had he expected? Should she have jumped into his arms and declared her love for him? He reminded himself what she'd said to him before he was supposed to go to Paris: *This is never going to happen.*

He just didn't believe her.

Moreover, he'd done some snooping into Jaiveer Babu last night. There wasn't much information about him on the Internet, but it did say that he came from Bengaluru, not Mumbai. Surely, if he and Francesca had been dating for a whole month, she would know where he came from.

Also, a lot of articles suggested Jaiveer was gay.

Which begged the same question as before: why was she lying to him?

He'd be talking to her about it later, whether she liked it or not. But right now, they had a wedding to shoot.

They parked the van with the other service providers and unloaded onto the pavement. Blenheim Palace was a great, hulking estate, the grandest of the grand country houses of England and bigger than Buckingham Palace. The main house faced onto a large courtyard, pillared porticos on either side forming a giant U. The grounds covered 2100 acres with grass, lakes, mazes and gardens. And people actually lived there! The Duke and Duchess of Marlborough owned the estate and still used it as their country bolt hole despite the non-stop tours and events that took place there. Krish had shot at Blenheim previously with Connor, but this was the first time that a client had rented the entire property, including the owners' private apartments. All tours today were cancelled.

With the heat and the scope of this wedding, it would be an exhausting day.

A staff member who introduced himself as Albert showed them to their breakout room, the same room where the downstairs servants usually took their meals while at work.

Albert, dressed in a three-piece dark suit with tails, explained that each member of their party would have a minder to shadow them when they worked in the private apartments above. He said this with a sharp, disdainful glance at Wally, who was running his finger up and down the Death tattoo on his neck. Krish was 99% sure he was doing it to freak out the officious staff member.

'And, for the love of King and country, don't sit on *anything* in the house,' instructed Albert. 'All the chairs and sofas are original antiques. If you damage anything...well, I hope you have *good* public liability insurance.'

The schedule up until the ceremony was vicious. First, bridal party photos in the garden; then Francesca and Stella would photograph the ceremony set-up before joining the bride in her boudoir upstairs. Meanwhile, Krish and Wally would cover the Baraat, where Paramjeet would process up the drive on a horse, accompanied by music and dancing. David would come with them to get overhead shots on his drone.

For a moment, Krish was struck by the enormity of the occasion. His first big event. Hopefully, it would be just the first in a long line of luxury bookings for Kapadia Photo/Video. He surveyed the room, where each member of the team was prepping equipment like the pros they were. David's allergies seemed to have settled for now. Wally wore red plaid trousers and a white t-shirt with a black bowtie printed at the neck, which Krish suspected was as fancy as Wally got.

Stella, always on point, had dressed in a sleeveless, belted dress patterned with lemons.

His gaze came to rest on Francesca in another Indian-style outfit, an aquamarine blue this time, a great colour that brought out her green eyes. He appreciated the effort to which she'd gone to look the part at this wedding. His heart unexpectedly swelled, and he turned away before she could catch the look on his face. A sudden image came to him of Francesca dressed in a red lehenga, her arms covered in henna, a red veil draped over her head.

The clock on the wall said 8:30. 'Right, team!' he called. 'Let's get wired up.' He brought out the box of headpieces, and they all chose one. He'd forgotten to mark which set had the faulty button, but he couldn't worry about that now.

He studied the map of the palace and asked Albert to show them to the garden at the west of the property.

Show time.

FRANCESCA WIPED THE SWEAT OFF HER FOREHEAD FOR THE HUNDREDTH time. She may have been hot, but at least she wasn't in pain. Like clockwork, her period and her symptoms had disappeared overnight. She felt like a normal human being again.

A really hot and sweaty normal human being.

It was almost 11:30, and the bride would arrive at the ceremony soon.

She took in the grandeur of the setting. The ceremony would take place outside, in a gigantic courtyard in front of the main entrance to the palace. Warm stone porticos with statues of women pointing at things sandwiched the space on opposite sides. Behind them was an open, grass-covered avenue that led up to a solitary column with a lonely figure on top.

The event planners had gone full Bollywood with the design. Real palm trees edged the seating area, and sheets of exotic flowers dangled between them, blocking the view of the actual palace the couple had paid an exorbitant fee to hire. A large, rounded Mandap on a platform dominated the front of the space, decked out in over-sized monstera leaves and flower arrangements in different shades of pink. A floral chandelier hung from the roof of the structure, suspended above plush, gilded Louis XIV-style armchairs. The ceremony would take place here. Real grass carpeted the Mandap.

Heat sizzled through the air, promising a sweaty day for everyone. Over the guests' heads, large, protective sails had been erected that stretched to the back of the courtyard. More flowers snaked up the poles holding the sails in place. Poor David had already started sneezing again.

Francesca had never seen an event design like it. She couldn't believe that Ishani and Paramjeet considered this their 'small' wedding.

The guests came prepared for a long, hot ceremony. Some held battery-operated fans. One lady brought binoculars to get a better view of the proceedings. Another aunty at the back unpacked a picnic basket full of food and served portions to the people sitting around her. Quite a few of the oldies were already taking naps. Or they had died. Francesca hoped for the former.

Paramjeet sat under the Mandap, along with both sets of parents. Francesca trained her lens on the groom's father, the famous director Vashney Oberoi, identifiable by his iconic black, fluffy eyebrows. A coronet of grey hair circled his head, leaving the top of his scalp bald as a baby. He was taller than she'd expected. She didn't get star struck as a rule, but a frisson of giddiness had shivered through her earlier when miking him up. He seemed nice, which made her wonder how he'd brought up such a wanker as Paramjeet.

At present, they were performing Hindu rituals before the bride arrived. Krish had warned her to expect a lot of rituals. He also said you never knew which rituals they would do, because it wasn't like the weddings she was used to, where things tended to happen the same way at every ceremony. At Hindu weddings, rituals were like a pick'n'mix, and no two Hindu weddings would ever be the same.

Briefly, she speculated about whether Krish would want an Indian wedding and which traditions he would choose to uphold. Her vision blurred, and for a moment she saw Krish and not Paramjeet under the Mandap. A mirage. She blinked her eyes a few times to dispel it.

The five hundred guests were seated now. Francesca spotted Jaiveer among them and waved. The ceremony would last two hours, followed by family photos on the steps of the palace. Just the expectation of everything they had left to do today made her crave bed.

Still, she was grateful. Because working kept her mind off Krish —and the fact that he wasn't engaged.

Her eyes wandered in his direction. They were covering close-ups while Wally and Stella shot wide. When Krish had appeared at breakfast that morning, she'd been surprised to see him in a short, tailored kurta instead of his usual suit. The top was royal blue linen with embroidery along the neckline and front and, on his bottom half, he wore camel-coloured pyjama-style trousers.

She bit her lip.

His shirt sleeves were pushed up, baring his forearms. The slim tailoring emphasised his trim, fit build. It was doing terrible things to her concentration.

Nope. She couldn't think about that now. She dragged her attention back to the Mandap.

The bride arrived under a moving canopy of flowers, a pole at each corner carried by four of the groomsmen. Ishani barely resembled herself underneath all her clothes, jewellery, and eyeliner. Deep red and edged with gold, her dress came in two parts: a cropped top baring a good deal of her flat stomach and a full, floor-length skirt that managed to appear light despite being covered in gold embroidery and jewels. A sheer red veil was attached to the back of her head, and an ornate diamanté choker necklace encircled her throat, finished off by two strings of fat pearls hanging between her breasts. And that was only half the jewellery. Dangling earrings weighed down her lobes, and her wrists clacked with bangles. A golden chain attached a nose ring to her ear. An Indian princess in the flesh. Francesca thought she had never seen such a gorgeous bride.

*What if I could be that bride?*

The intrusive thought almost made her drop her camera.

For a moment, she allowed herself to fantasise, to pretend it was her wearing the red lehenga and Krish waiting for her, shoeless, under the Mandap.

The idea of it glowed through her.

*Tell him!* yelled King Rat in her head. She commanded her inner rodent to shut up. And at what point did she need to start worrying that she had imaginary conversations with a rat?

*You've built a cage.* Jaiveer's proclamation came hot on the heels of King Rat.

That damned cage...

That cage was a story she told herself about her pain. About what would happen if she opened up about it. She'd spent her whole lifetime building it. What if she was wrong?

Would she let fear continue to control her life? What if she just... didn't? What if she decided to love herself? What if she *could* be that bride? What if Krish *did* choose her? And more importantly, what if *she* chose *Krish*?

If there was one man in the world who might accept her exactly the way she was, it was Krish. His kindness, his strength, especially his Lancelot Complex...he was the best of men. She had never met anyone else like him. The Universe had tried to push him into her path five years ago, but she had been too stupid and too cynical and too full of self-loathing to believe her luck.

*The only thing standing between you and the life you want is yourself.* The realisation made her breath catch.

As the bride and groom started walking around the fire in the centre of the Mandap, Francesca raised her eyes from her viewfinder to locate Krish. He was hunched on the steps of the Mandap, camera in hand, only ten feet away.

*Look at me. Look at me. Look at me.* She willed it with her entire being.

He continued to focus on the ceremony. Francesca imagined she could feel the heat from the fire on her skin.

*If he looks at me now, then I'll never tell another lie again,* she prayed to whomever was listening.

And then, like a miracle, Krish turned his head towards her.

Their gazes locked.

Everything else disappeared: the guests, the palm trees, the couple. It all faded to white as she stared at him. At the face she loved.

For the first time, she let him see that she cared about him with all her heart. Her eyes softened. She parted her lips, and her breathing sped up. Her breasts heaved with desire, and a delicious ache began in her very core. She let everything go.

He narrowed his eyes, and his tongue darted out to lick his lips.

If there hadn't been five hundred people watching, she would have leapt on him and had him in the central aisle.

The audience applauded.

Both of them shook their heads, re-engaging with the ceremony.

Inside, she buzzed with excitement.

This was happening.

*This was happening.*

KRISH DIDN'T KNOW WHAT IT WAS, BUT SOMETHING HAD SHIFTED between him and Francesca. The way she looked at him during the Saptapadi...

...If eyes could shag.

He couldn't remember why he'd followed the urge to look at her at that exact point in the ceremony, when the bride and groom swapped places in their journey around the holy fire of Agni. It was called the Seven Steps. The first four times, the man walked in front, tugging his bride by the pinky; then the last three turns, they switched places, all while the pandit chanted the seven promises. The Fire God Agni bore witness to this, the most sacred part of the ceremony.

A voice inside had told him to look up, so he had.

He found her staring at him openly, in a way she had never done in the past. Everything was written on her face.

She loved him.

He didn't need to hear her say it. He could see it. It was in her eyes. They radiated yearning, unblinking, possessing him. Together, he and Francesca were absorbed in a mutual trance.

If the Fire God was present in that moment, Krish wouldn't have been surprised.

When the audience had started clapping at the end of the ritual, the sudden loss of that connection made him dizzy. It took him a moment to remember he was supposed to be taking pictures.

The rest of the wedding felt like foreplay.

During the drinks reception in the Long Library, they stood next to each other in front of an imposing alabaster statue of Queen Ann. 'Oh my god,' she said in an excited whisper, 'is that Katrina Kaif?'

'How do you know who Katrina Kaif is?' She was a Bollywood star famous for her dancing skills.

'*Bang Bang? Baar Baar Dekho?*'

'I didn't know you were such a Hindi film aficionado.'

'There's a lot you don't know about me, Kapadia.' She gave him a mysterious half smile and looked away.

He laughed and shook his head. She was finally opening up to him, and it made him happy. They continued to stand next to each other for a few more minutes, even though they probably should have been moving through the crowd.

Her presence felt more solid and real than anything else in the room. The books, the guests getting drunk on expensive champagne, the unexpected, imposing pipe organ at the other end of the room. All of these things seemed like ghosts in a reality where only he existed with Francesca. Their cameras hung around their necks, dormant. He turned his head away from her, afraid that if he started gazing into her eyes, he wouldn't be able to stop. Instead, his fingers fluttered towards hers. Her pinky brushed against his, and that small touch was everything.

The contact sent an electric shock through his body. He could feel himself growing hard with anticipation, a bad idea in these loose trousers. With reluctance, he broke away, turned towards the wall and found sudden interest in photographing the carved ceiling.

All he desired was to find a moment alone to kiss her. That could sustain him until later, when he planned to show her just how much he'd wanted her these past few weeks. The day had been tiring, but he was sure he could squirrel away a parcel of energy for that.

The wedding, which had seemed to fly by in the beginning, now dragged with the weight of expectation. He thought he might get a moment with her during their lunch break, but the team ended up eating at different times. Then there were more family photos, more outfit changes, more cocktails on the lawn.

Finally, many hours later, the moment arrived after they'd photographed the couple, and Paramjeet and Ishani returned to their chambers for a half hour alone before the final push. The evening guests had arrived and were finding their seats in the massive marquee on the south lawn, where the meal would be served in an hour and the evening's entertainment would take place. For the first time that day, nothing needed filming or photographing .

'I forgot something in the library. Back in a minute. Over,' Francesca's voice said through the earpiece.

She didn't have to tell him twice. He knew she was talking just to him.

From the door of the marquee, he saw her heading up the stairs to the palace, and he followed. Just before she disappeared into the building, she stopped and glanced over her shoulder, as though checking he'd gotten the message. He caught up with her as she was walking down the long corridor, portraits of Georgian dukes and duchesses watching on. 'Francesca!' he called out.

She stopped and turned towards him with a brazen grin.

They stood facing each other, both of them taking shallow breaths, like air was in short supply.

Searching her eyes, he asked, 'Have I read things wrong? Or—'

'No,' she whispered, placing her palm against the centre of his chest and fingering the embroidery there.

'Thank fuck for that.' Not wanting to rush the moment, he raised his hands to frame her face, stroking the top of her cheekbones with his thumbs.

She shivered and closed her eyes.

Slowly, he bent his lips towards hers. Her breath tickled the bare skin where his beard used to be.

'Surprise, Little!' screeched a voice behind him. 'I've been looking everywhere for you.'

*No, it couldn't be...*

He muttered a silent curse. Imaginary cold water doused his passion. Gazing down at Francesca's confused face, he said, 'I'm sorry.'

And then he spun around.

FRANCESCA HAD NO IDEA WHAT WAS GOING ON. ONE SECOND, ALL OF her Christmases were about to come at once, and then bang! Gone! Krish apologised—for what, she didn't know—and turned away from her.

And was she crazy, or was he trying to shield her from the interloper with his body? His hands were on his hips, his elbows flapped out like elephant ears, as though trying to make himself a bigger barrier. She stepped swiftly to the right to unmask the stranger's identity.

Ankita, Krish's sister, stood a few feet away, her neat baby bump hugged by a shimmering silver dress. Glossy, pregnancy-enhanced black hair hung loose over her shoulder. Ankita had always been glamorous; Francesca had never seen her without full make-up.

When Krish and Francesca were dating, she and Krish's sister had gotten on well—better than Francesca got on with her own sister, anyway. The years had dulled her memory of Ankita's voice, but now she remembered their Big/Little nickname thing.

Francesca smiled and opened her mouth to say hello.

Ankita jumped in first. 'What the hell is *she* doing here?'

It took Francesca a moment to realise Ankita was talking about *her*.

'She's filming the wedding. What are *you* doing here?' countered Krish.

Using the petite black designer clutch in her hand to gesticulate in the general direction of the wedding, Ankita snapped, 'Who do you think got you this job? I know Ishani through work.'

'Why didn't you tell me?'

'Because I wanted to surprise you, dummy. Must say, I'm the one who's surprised.'

'It's not what you think.' He took a step towards his sister, further away from Francesca.

*What did he mean by that?* Was he disavowing her before they'd even reconciled?

Ankita put a hand on her waist and poked Krish in the chest with her clutch. 'Does Jess know about this?'

'Jess and I broke up.'

Her mouth fell open. 'What?! I thought you were going to propose in Paris...'

Krish held his arms out wide. 'Well, I didn't.'

'Because of *her*?' Ankita said, scowling at Francesca.

'No, because of *me*.'

Ankita put a hand on her bump and took an uncertain step to the side. 'I think I need to sit down.' She looked around for somewhere to park herself, but all the chairs were behind ropes, with signs that read 'Do not sit'.

'Big! You okay?' He reached towards her while simultaneously swinging his head left and right, looking for a chair alternative.

There were none. To Francesca he said, 'Can you please stay with her? I'm going to find something for her to sit on.'

Without hesitation, Francesca did as he asked. She stood awkwardly near Ankita, ready to catch her at any moment. It smarted to realise that somebody she'd had warm memories of all these years hated her. But it made sense. Of course Ankita hated her. Francesca's head must have been fuzzy with passion to think otherwise.

As soon as Krish left, his sister dropped her hand, stood up straight, and turned on Francesca. She pointed her clutch like a sword at Francesca. 'Listen. I don't know how you ended up here, but you broke his heart once, and *I* was the one who had to deal with it. He loved you, and you just dumped him for some other man.'

'I know that's what it looked like, but—'

'Bup. Bup.' Ankita held up her free hand and tapped her fingers against her thumb like the mouth of a puppet snapping shut. 'I don't care what you have to say. His life was finally back on track. It took two years for him to get over you. *Two years!*' She practically spat those words. 'Jess was *perfect* for him. I introduced them myself.'

Francesca was speechless. Her newfound confidence withered. If Ankita hated her this much, then what about Krish's parents? They probably hated her, too. She remembered Sunday lunches at their house: the intelligent discussions, the laughter, the love around the table—so different to her own family gatherings, where she never belonged. Krish's parents had always made her believe she was one of the family. How would they take the news that she and Krish were back together? Would they be able to forgive her? Or would she be condemning them all to a lifetime of tolerating her at family get-togethers? And what would they think when they found out Francesca couldn't give them grandkids?

King Rat's decide-to-love-yourself pep talk grew muted as Francesca returned to familiar ground. She'd caused Krish so much pain. Being with her would only cause him more. She lowered her eyes, crossing her arms over her stomach.

'If you cared for him at all,' Ankita continued, 'then you'd disappear from his life again and let him patch things up with Jess. You are no good for him.'

The doors behind them burst open, and Krish came through carrying a chair. A blonde, tall man in a tuxedo followed him. Francesca recognised Ankita's husband, although his name escaped her.

'Kiki, are you okay? The baby…' he said.

Krish put the chair down, but Ankita didn't sit. 'I'm fine, fine.' She waved him away.

Stella's voice sounded in their earpieces. 'Bride and groom arriving soon. Where is everybody? Over.'

Krish ran his hands through his hair, obviously conflicted about what to do. 'We've got to get back to work. Max, can I leave her with you?'

'Of course. Go. We'll be fine.'

'Francesca?' Krish jerked his head towards the door and held his hand out to her.

'Oh…um….' Why had she been walking towards the library again? Oh, yeah. Her lens cap. She had actually left it on the base of the Queen Ann statue and was going back to retrieve it. 'I'll…um… join you in a moment. I forgot something in the other room.' Without waiting for a reply, she turned on her heel and jogged down the corridor, tears running down her cheeks.

# 26

FRANCESCA WENT through the motions of filming the wedding. She barely noticed what was happening. Some speeches. Some laughter. People being happy.

She was numb to it all.

Even Jaiveer's dance extravaganza failed to shake her from her daze. Normally, she would have loved something like that: a live Bollywood number by an award-winning choreographer with Katrina Kaif as a surprise guest...Francesca should have been whooping along and wiggling her hips.

But she stood still, staring through her screen at the twirling, gyrating, thrusting dancers, vacuuming up footage with her camera, not registering what was going on.

Was Ankita right?

With Jess, Krish had a good thing going, and then along came Hurricane Francesca, wiping out everything in her wake. Just like her family always said. Perhaps she wasn't meant to be the heroine in this Bollywood film, but the villain.

Five years ago, she had broken Krish's heart. Hers didn't come out unscathed either, but she still remembered the look on his face when she said she was dating someone else.

Pain. Like she had reached into his chest and squeezed his heart to a pulp.

Being so close to him these past few weeks, she'd become disoriented and lost sight of the reason she'd walked away from him in the first place: she could not give him what he wanted.

She was broken. And he had no idea.

He was falling in love with an illusion.

Pressing the button on her mic, she said, 'Wally, can you cover the bride and groom for a minute? Over.'

'Righty-ho. Over.'

Hidden behind the speakers, she dropped her head into her hands. Her determination to tell Krish everything wavered and fear gripped her. Her worst qualities spooled through her mind on a familiar loop: *you're sick, you're a drain, you're antisocial, nobody likes you, you don't deserve to be happy.*

She hit her palm against her forehead. *Shut the fuck up*, she told that voice. After her chat with the rat, she had realised that the negative voice wasn't really hers. It was the voice of the saboteur who lived inside her. She'd even given it a name: Cynthia, after the receptionist at her GP's office who always looked at Francesca funny when she came into the surgery. Cynthia was a bitch.

Unfortunately, Ankita and Cynthia seemed to be on the same page. Francesca wiped the tears off her face.

She had to get a fucking grip. The tired old record in her head was wearing thin. Cynthia needed to go on a permanent holiday. Closing her eyes, she tried to regain some of the self-love that she'd felt so strongly during the ceremony, when she'd opened herself up to Krish's gaze and showed him her very soul.

'Goldie! What are you doing back here?' Jaiveer was walking past, pulling one of the other male dancers behind him. They were both still sweaty after the big number. Francesca suspected they were on their way to get even more sweaty.

He murmured something to his friend, who sashayed back to the dance floor. Jaiveer grabbed her hand and pulled her outside the marquee into the cool night air. He peeled his jacket off and fanned himself. The male dancers had all worn fitted suits, like in the famous reunion scene in *Yeh Jawaani Hai Deewani*, except Jaiveer's suit was bright pink and sequinned.

'Great job on the dance,' she said, even though she couldn't remember it.

'Thanks. Glad it's over,' he confided. 'Now, tell me why you were hiding behind a speaker crying?'

She groaned. 'His sister is here. She said all kinds of awful things to me and…well…now I'm scared to tell him…you know.'

He took her by the shoulders. 'We talked about this. The cage…'

'The fucking cage. Blah blah blah.'

He tilted his head to the side, like a know-it-all. 'You need to tell him.'

'I know that! I'm just not sure *how*.'

'You'll figure something out.' He picked a piece of thread off her shirt and pulled her in for a hug.

She let her head sink onto his chest. Thankfully, his shirt had dried. 'I was so naive to think we could just pick up where we left off. What if his family can't forgive me…?'

Stroking the back of her head, Jaiveer said, 'You aren't dating his family. And you won't be picking up where you left off. You'll be starting over again. With *no secrets* between you.'

Francesca was about to respond when Krish's voice crackled over the headphones. 'Um, Francesca? We can all hear you.' A beat. 'Over.'

With wide, terrified eyes, she stepped out of Jaiveer's arms and tented her hands over her mouth. 'Oh my god.'

She had the faulty headset.

*Bollocks.*

Clicking the button again, she tore the mic from her collar, just to make sure it was off.

'What's wrong?' asked Jaiveer. He grasped her by the hand. 'Goldie, what's wrong? You look ill.'

And even though he was inside the tent and she was outside of it

251

and he probably couldn't see her, she could feel Krish's eyes piercing her like daggers. Her throat constricted, and she struggled to speak. 'He heard me,' she whispered hoarsely. 'He heard everything we just said.'

'Oooh,' said Jaiveer, wincing. 'Well, as my grandmother used to say: *to control the mind is like trying to control a drunken monkey that has been bitten by a scorpion.*'

'What the fuck does that mean?'

'No idea. She usually said it whenever I was being stupid about something.' He shrugged and patted her twice on the cheek. 'Just tell him.'

She would have liked more sympathy.

'Okay, team,' Krish announced through the headset. 'We still have a couple more hours on the clock. Let's just get through those and... and, Francesca, we'll talk later. Over.'

*Over.* That one word said so much.

## 27

FOR THE REST of the wedding, Francesca kept herself busy by cataloguing female villains. Cruella DeVille, animal cruelty at its finest. Nurse Ratched, who should have thought twice about her job choice. Bellatrix LeStrange, so terrifying she made Voldemort look like a puppy. Francesca March, liar and heartbreaker extraordinaire.

When she tired of that, she played word games. Could she come up with a different word for 'idiot' with each letter of the alphabet?

*Arsehole, bonehead, clod, dipshit, eejit, Francesca...*

Anything—she'd rather think of *anything* than the storm that was coming.

Jaiveer, taking the role of new friend very seriously, offered to get her drunk, but she explained that she still had work to do, tempting as the offer was. After extracting a promise from her to text him later with any news, he went in search of the dancing boy from earlier.

The worst thing was Krish's silence.

He hadn't said two words to her since Mic-gate.

Unless she counted: 'Start taking the bags to the van' when they finished shooting and he returned to the marquee to say goodbye to Ankita and her husband.

Inside, dread unfurled, one capillary at a time. No hiding anymore. But old habits died hard and hiding was *all* she wanted to do. The urge to run off into the grounds of Blenheim and disappear into the night like Cathy on the moors seemed like a feasible idea. She could pass into local legend, and they could talk about her on the tours, calling her the 'Crazy Lady of Blenheim' and recounting how they could still hear her desperate voice crackling through microphones on certain wedding nights: *'Can you keep a secret, my precioussssss?'*

She'd had worse ideas.

Her back resting on the van, she dropped her head into her hands and shook it back and forth. No. It was time to stop running. She'd have to tell him all her secrets now, including the one about Norman.

As he walked past, Wally stopped to punch her on the arm in encouragement. 'Good luck, mate,' he said.

David couldn't even look at her. His face was red by association, as though vicariously living the embarrassment with her.

Stella gave her a motherly hug, which Francesca tolerated.

'I don't know what's going on between you,' Stella said, 'but I know you'll work it out.'

A sob caught in Francesca's throat and she pressed it back down.

Nobody spoke on the way to the B&B. Francesca could just imagine the tennis game of significant looks playing in the van. She couldn't see them, as she'd slipped into the back seat and was lying across it. She stared up into the inky night sky, the occasional street lamp blinding her as they zoomed past.

When they pulled into the drive, she grabbed her camera bag and sprinted for the front door, thinking that if she could barricade herself in her room, she could push this conversation back another 24 hours. Safely behind her locked door, she listened for footsteps. One, two, three, four doors shutting. She waited, counting the footballs on the wallpaper. Thirty-six. They floated on a deep blue background. A cherry red Arsenal duvet set covered the single bed, which was pushed up against the wall in the corner. Luckily, despite it being a child's room, there was an en-suite bathroom. Wanting to shed every reminder of today, she peeled off her aquamarine outfit and jumped into the shower, washing her hair twice for good measure (and to take up time).

As she collapsed onto the bed with the wet towel still wrapped around her and damp hair hanging around her shoulders, she allowed herself to relax, thinking she had evaded Krish for yet another day.

Knock. Knock. Knock.

She bolted upright. *Oh, shit.*

What was she going to say? She had been in denial about the whole awful affair and hadn't rehearsed anything. She pulled the towel over her face, like a child hiding behind a skinny tree.

The knock came again. 'Francesca. Open the door, or I'm going to break it down.'

*Right then.* 'Hold your horses,' she said to mollify him. She took a deep breath and pushed herself off the bed. She couldn't answer the door in a towel. Fortunately, a fluffy white robe hung on the side of the IKEA wardrobe. Unfortunately, it had black Friesian spots all over and cow horns sprouting from the hood. It was about two sizes too big, but it would have to do.

Belting it on, she gripped the door handle and ripped it open, like removing a plaster.

Krish didn't wait to be invited in. The room immediately filled with his presence. He had changed too, into loose blue cotton pyjama bottoms and a white t-shirt. His hair was damp, the sweet smell of his shampoo wafting past her nose.

How did one behave in this sort of scenario? 'Drink?' she offered, waving her hand towards her tea and coffee making facilities.

'I'm fine, thanks.' Always polite.

'Okay, then. What can I do for you at one in the morning?'

'You know why I'm here.' He stood in the middle of the room, crossed his arms, and probed her with his dark eyes. 'Francesca, what's going on?'

She just shrugged and studied the floor, too many words crowding her mouth.

'Just tell me. No more secrets.'

A quick glance at him revealed an angry vein throbbing on his neck, belying the controlled calm in his voice. She couldn't do this. She pulled the hood of her robe over her head to hide in plain sight.

He reached out and grasped one of the horns on the hood, tugging it back down again. 'Okay, okay,' he said, like he was trying to reason with a wild animal. 'Let's start with this: why did you lie to me about Jaiveer? You two obviously weren't dating.'

Francesca blew out a stuttering breath, grateful that even through his anger, he knew that asking her specific questions would make it easier for her to answer. *Here goes nothing.* 'Because Ankita was right. I'm no good for you.'

'Did she say that?'

Her eyes grew moist and she nodded.

He threw his hands up in the air. 'She doesn't know anything,' he said. 'She doesn't understand...this. All she knows is what happened...'

She heard the part he didn't say: 'When you broke my heart.' A tear slid down her cheek and he took a step towards her, wiping it away with the pad of this thumb. She would have loved it if he took her into his arms so she could bury her head against his body, hide herself in him. But he didn't. He stood in front of her, close enough that she could feel the heat from him but without letting her hide. He tilted her chin up towards him.

'Chezzy. Look at me. Please. I need to know...what's so terrible you had to keep it from me?' His voice caught on the last word.

She opened her mouth, but nothing came out.

Taking her by surprise, his hands gripped her upper arms. Heat rushed to his touch. The only thing holding her up right now were those hands. 'I've spent five years wracking my brains, replaying our whole relationship, trying to figure out what happened. One minute we were happy, and the next—poof—you were gone.' The volume of his voice rose as he spoke. 'Just tell me.'

The pressure of keeping the truth from him shattered her. The words began in her belly and travelled up her throat, battering down her usual barriers. Finally, she erupted: 'I can't have children, Krish!'

As soon as it was out of her mouth, her whole body slumped, as though the secret had been her life-support. She cried out. Krish caught her and picked her up like a rag doll, depositing her on the edge of the bed. He kneeled on the floor in front of her, supporting her head between his large hands.

She gripped the edge of the duvet, trembling, shocked that the truth was out in the wild. She could probably fly if she flapped her arms—she felt that light. Another sensation flowed through her, and she was surprised to identify it as...relief?

Encouraging her to look into his eyes and failing, he begged, 'Tell me what you mean.'

'I mean I can't have children. Like, *ever*. I'm broken.'

'What?'

'I've got everything. Polycystic ovaries, fibroids, endometriosis... and zero fertility.'

'That's it?' he asked with incredulity. He let go of her head and sat back on his heels.

'What do you mean "that's it"? That's *a lot*.' She concentrated on balling up the ends of her bathrobe's belt.

Krish shifted into a more comfortable position, leaning his elbow onto his knee. 'So let me get this straight. Instead of telling me all of this five years ago, you broke up with me?'

She nodded.

'And Norman...?'

The ball she'd made out of the belt unfurled as soon as she let it go. 'I made him up.'

He snapped his fingers. 'I knew it!'

257

'You did?' Francesca peeked at him through her curtain of wet hair.

'Yes, I mean…Norman? I just couldn't picture you falling for a Norman.'

He had a point. Apologies to the Normans of the world.

'All this time,' he said, looking up as though replaying a slideshow in his head, 'all this time, I thought I'd done something wrong. Maybe I spooked you by saying "I love you" too soon in Paris. Or I got too intense. Maybe I was bad in bed.' He shook his head and ran his hand through his wet hair.

'Well you know that's not true,' she said, wiping more tears from her face.

'You bloody fool.' He turned his gaze on her. 'You thought I would leave you if I knew?'

She both nodded and whispered, 'Yes.'

Francesca watched his pupils darken, the smile falling from his face. Delicately, he pushed the robe off her knees, exposing bare skin. For a moment, his thumbs made lazy circles on the sensitive spot right on top of the joint.

'Just so you know, we're going to talk more about this later. But right now, I don't want to talk. Is that okay?' He bent down and placed a soft, butterfly kiss on the inside of her knee.

Was that okay? Was water wet? God knew she was. She bit her lip and nodded. The tiredness from the past two days disappeared. Adrenaline snaked through her veins, lighting her up. Heat gathered in her core. She was filled with lava, a volcano about to explode. All she wanted to do was kiss him, but when she leaned towards him, he leaned back with a mischievous grin, those sexy dimples denting his cheeks. She wanted to lick them.

Krish slowly pushed open her knees so that her legs splayed wide and slid his own body close to hers, stomach to stomach. The rough string bow on the waistband of his pyjamas brushed her most sensitive spot, and she almost came then and there. She caught her breath. The air in the room stilled, and quiet static filled her ears.

He didn't kiss her, but she could feel his lips near her neck, as though he held a smouldering coal inches from her skin. He hovered at her temple, her ear, the place where neck met shoulder—not touching, just letting the heat from his breath bring up goosebumps. He remembered exactly how to drive her wild.

She couldn't believe she was here. With Krish. *Her* Krish. The spark inside her that had ignited when she was 'speaking' with the rat grew brighter. This was what she'd been chasing since she left him all those years ago. This utter and complete feeling of self-acceptance. Of surrender. Of wanting to belong to one person. Of connection that she had never achieved with anyone else. Francesca was his to do with as he wanted.

Reaching down, he untied the belt holding her robe closed. It took ages, although it was probably only a few seconds. With maddening slowness, he slithered the robe off her shoulders, exposing all of her to his gaze. Her nipples hardened.

All she desired was for him to take them in his mouth, but he didn't. He just soaked her in with his eyes.

'Fucking hell, I've missed the sight of you. You're so beautiful,' he said. Those words made the light inside her grow even bigger.

She freed her arms from the robe's sleeves and leaned back on her elbows, so he could see all of her. Her breasts grew heavy with desire. The urge to wrap her legs around him and grind him into her...it would be so easy. But she waited because she knew it was what he required of her. She whimpered.

'Lie down,' he commanded. She loved it when he got bossy.

Francesca dropped back onto the bed, wet hair squishing underneath her shoulders. Anticipation made her entire body tighten with need. Every inch of her skin was caressed by the warm air, but fuck the air. She wanted Krish to touch her. She reached to pull him closer and he caught first one and then the other wrist, pressing them down into the bed.

He bent over her. The delicate flick of his tongue on the inside of her thigh was so light she wasn't sure she'd actually felt it.

'Please,' she begged.

His tongue got to work, licking and tickling, everywhere except where she actually wanted it. She'd forgotten just how good he was, almost like he'd studied how to pleasure a woman. He'd always been an A+ student. She imagined him making notes in his meticulous hand, fingers tracing the shape of the female clitoris, a big arrow pointing to the nub, saying 'Orgasm here.' She was loving his commitment.

Krish let go of her hands so he could stroke the skin on her inner thigh, increasing her anticipation. One of her freed hands flew to her breast, the other to his head. She swallowed hard and urged him higher.

He pushed her knees further apart. Krish looked up at her and smirked, a wicked glint in his eye. Yes, he knew exactly what he was doing. With his thumbs, he stretched the skin on either side of her vulva wide and gently touched the middle with his tongue.

She screamed.

Wrapping her legs around his shoulders, she squeezed his head as she rode the orgasm she'd wanted for five years. 'Krish!'

He licked her one last time and kissed the inside of her thigh, like his work there was done for now.

But hers wasn't.

The aftermath of her pleasure still flowing through her, Francesca sat up, forcing him upright, too. Taking his head between her hands, she pulled his lips to hers, tasting the sweetness of herself there. Her hands wandered down his back and gathered his shirt. He got the hint, pulling away a moment to divest himself of it. Standing, he pushed his trousers down, his massive penis bouncing into view. She'd forgotten how big he was. Exactly in proportion to the rest of him.

She grasped him in her hand and licked the tip. 'Do you want...?' she asked.

'No. I've waited so long. I just want to be inside you.' He could barely get the words out.

Who was she to argue?

She pushed him down onto the single bed and straddled him. Usually at this point, she'd insist on a condom, but she knew this man. He was *her* Krish. He was trustworthy and kind and caring and, most importantly, careful. And there was no danger of getting pregnant.

'Are you ready?' she asked with a crooked smile, enjoying the total and utter need on his face.

He nodded. His eyes glazed.

She positioned herself above him, enjoying the sensation of rubbing against him and watching him shudder with raging desire. Two could play the delayed gratification game. She rested her free hand on top of his heart, letting it beat through her like an ultrasound.

'Please,' he begged.

'Say my name,' she commanded, loving the wiry feel of his chest hairs between her fingers.

'Francesca.' It sounded delicious coming from his mouth, his voice. She had dreamed of that voice. She could bathe in that voice.

Taking mercy on them both, she slid her body onto him, filling the cavity that she'd self-inflicted five years ago. It was like she'd been made for him, and he for her. How could she ever have doubted that?

As they chased climax, she imagined the light that had been growing inside her, bursting out of her mouth, her eyes, her ears, her fingers.

She loved Krish. She loved herself.

*The rest will follow.*

## 28

KRISH SMILED. He couldn't help it. It had been the most amazing night since...well...five years ago.

The bed was small. His feet stuck off the bottom edge. He was wrapped in an Arsenal duvet, despite being a Man U fan.

But it was perfect.

He might even look upon Arsenal with fondness from now on.

Funny how memory worked. There were so many things that had stuck in his head over the years, like the squeaking noise she made when she orgasmed and the mole on her left breast. But for every detail he remembered, there was something that had grown fuzzy with time: how she bucked when he sucked on her nipples. The exact taste of her in his mouth, like peaches. Memory definitely didn't do these things justice.

He nuzzled Francesca's neck, and she sighed. They laid together on the single bed like two puzzle pieces, her back to him, body mirroring his. He ran his hand over the curve of her hips. How he loved those curves. How he had missed the way she looked at him, like he belonged to her. How he craved making love with her. It always felt like more than a tangle of bodies; it was a meeting of minds. His body responded immediately, but he breathed in and counted to five while his brain regained control. They needed to talk first, even though the clock was pushing 3AM.

Propping his head on his hand, he retreated towards the football-covered wall, giving her room to turn onto her back. He waited for her to get comfortable, to look at him with her clear green eyes. When he had been kissing her stomach, he'd noticed three small scars. Now he rubbed them with his thumb, delicately, reverentially.

'Those ones are from laser surgery,' she said, watching his hand. 'I've already had two rounds.'

Krish would have liked to kiss each one again, but the size of the bed prohibited it. 'I wish I could have been there for you.' He would be, next time she needed him.

She laughed, a short huff without any humour in it. 'Me, too.'

How brave she'd been to go through it all alone. 'So, tell me about it.'

Francesca turned her head away and closed her eyes. He waited for her to be ready. Krish was aware that this thing between them was still brittle, and he didn't want to scare her away.

Her lips in a small O, she pushed a string of air out, like she was blowing out a candle. Preparing herself. He snuggled closer, wanting to keep her safe.

'Remember how I used to pop ibuprofen like candy?' she said. 'How I sometimes cancelled dates at the last minute? And, you know, how I get a little cranky sometimes?'

The meeting with Paramjeet and Ishani popped into his head. Cranky? He nodded, also recalling how he'd commented on her pill popping way back when they were dating. 'You're going to end up with a hole in your stomach, if you're not careful,' he'd said, concerned because his mum had mentioned something about the side effects of excessive ibuprofen.

'Well, it was because I have all these reproductive problems. Polycystic ovaries, which make me break out and gain weight if I'm not constantly careful. Fibroids, which cause heavy bleeding and back ache. And endometriosis is the worst. It gives me stabbing pain. All the fucking time.'

Krish flinched, thinking about how much he hadn't known about her. How had he not noticed?

'Too much information?' she asked with a sad smile.

He pulled her into a tight hug. 'Not at all. You forget...I grew up in a house of women, so...'

'Yeah. I know.' She inhaled deeply and continued. 'The gyno told me it'd be unlikely that I'd be able to have children.'

'Unlikely? That's not 100%, then...' He tucked a piece of hair behind her ear and she turned away. *Shit.* He'd said the wrong thing.

'Krish, I'm a mess down there. Even if there were a chance, I don't think I'd want to risk it. Anyways...'

She grew silent and closed her eyes again.

'What?' He nudged her, willing her to speak.

Turning back towards him, she held his gaze, unblinking, as though about to give him a test. 'I'm scheduled to have a hysterectomy in October. It won't cure the endometriosis, but it will reduce the other symptoms.'

He hoped he managed to hide the flinch of shock that shot across his face.

'Krish!' Tears leaked from the corners of her eyes. 'I just *can't* anymore. I can't take it. I have to do it!'

'Shhhh.' He crushed her sobbing body to him and shushed until she calmed.

Meanwhile, his thoughts raced. A hysterectomy would be final. How did he feel about that? Obviously, it was her body, and she had complete control over what she did with it. But how did he feel about the thought of never having children with her? Maybe they could harvest some of her eggs before she did it. He'd look into it.

'I can tell it bothers you. I was right to leave.' She tried to pull away again, but he wouldn't let her. His arms tightened around her.

'That's not fair.' He kissed her ear. 'You need to give me a moment to digest this.'

Her body stilled, and she stopped trying to escape him. He rubbed his thumb over her belly. She said, 'You've always talked about having a big family.'

She was right. He couldn't remember the exact conversations, but he was sure he'd told her that. He thought of his sister, now in her last few weeks of pregnancy. Maybe it would be enough for Ankita to carry on the genetic line. He could still have a big family. If he wanted to be with Francesca, then they could give a loving home to other children who needed one.

'We could adopt,' he said, meaning it completely. He smiled like he had just solved all their problems.

Francesca shook her head. 'It's a possibility, but I'm worried that I'd be a crap mother. I've spent so many years telling myself that I'd never be one. *Accepting* that fact. I'd have to think about it.' Francesca faced her body towards him and stared into his eyes, brushing the hair off his forehead.

He could see the turmoil in her face. He wanted to make it all better for her. 'I'm here for you now, and I'm not going anywhere.' *I love you*, he thought, not yet ready to say it out loud. What if she walked away again? What if he still couldn't trust her? What if she broke his heart a second time? His preservation instinct counselled him towards caution, even as his body reacted to her.

With no more words, they made love again. This time slower. Afterwards, he stroked his hand up and down her spine, urging her to sleep. They both needed it. Eventually, he heard her slip into the rhythmic, even breathing of deep slumber. He wished he could do the same.

## 29

'SOMEBODY WAS HAVING FUN LAST NIGHT,' said the B&B host with a wide yawn as he delivered a fresh pot of coffee.

'Wasn't me!' Stella said with an uncomfortable smile. The last thing she wanted to do was discuss Krish and Francesca's orgasmic vocal range with a septuagenarian stranger. 'Is there any more brown sugar?'

'I'll get some,' he said. 'Don't worry—there's no hurry to check out. I don't have new guests coming until Tuesday.'

'Thanks,' she said. It was already eleven o'clock, and she was keen to get home. She had a husband to tell off.

Her anger at Connor had been simmering steadily for two days now. For the last hour, she'd passed the time by scrolling through photos on her phone from their trip abroad to remind herself that she loved him.

She *did* love Connor. But she was also really pissed off with him.

'Morning,' said Wally as he ambled into the sunny breakfast room with a chipper smile. 'Sleep okay?'

'Ummmmm...' She wrinkled her nose and shook her head. 'Not really. You?'

'Great! Like a baby.'

*You didn't have the room next to the Oxford Shag-a-thon,* she thought. She remembered the residential course she'd done in France with Connor, before they were together. On that trip, she'd also had the adjoining room to a horny couple. She wondered briefly what had happened to them. Were they still together? Then she realised she didn't care. They'd been vile.

But Francesca and Krish...she was happy they had sorted things out. Really happy. But also deeply, deeply tired.

'Good morning,' said David, as he walked in and went straight to the cereal bar. He poured himself a bowl of Coco Pops and sat at a different table from Stella and Wally.

'How are the allergies?' asked Stella with concern.

'Fine.' He shovelled a spoonful of cereal into his mouth. He obviously wasn't in a talkative mood today. Maybe they'd kept him up, too.

The stairs creaked, and Stella was surprised to see Francesca come in, freshly showered and lively. Stella thought they'd sleep in a bit more, especially since they'd been up until 3AM, and then at 5AM, and then again at 8AM...

'Hello, nerds!' Francesca greeted them all with a huge grin.

Lashings of sex seemed to agree with her. Stella had never seen her so jolly.

'Is there any oat milk?' Francesca asked the owner, who scurried back to the kitchen to find some.

David was eating Coco Pops like he might find the meaning of life at the bottom of his bowl.

'How are your allergies?' Francesca asked him.

He made a strangled noise, and Stella could see his cheeks reddening from where she sat. Poor boy had probably received a bit of an education last night. His room was directly above Francesca's.

'Good morning!' Krish bounded in last but not least. Stella had to admire their energy. They were probably still high on adrenaline and dopamine and whatever other feel-good body chemicals existed. She remembered the early days of her relationship with

Connor, when they could barely keep their hands off each other and he paid as much attention to her out of bed as in it. When had that started to change? She couldn't pinpoint an exact time. Had it been while they were travelling? Or before that, when she started stepping away from the business towards the end of her pregnancy?

All she knew was that she wanted things to get better again.

She watched Krish touch Francesca briefly on the lower back before helping himself to the croissants and melon. It was such a small gesture, but it spoke so loudly, possessive and protective at the same time.

Stella wondered exactly what had gone down in that room last night. Obviously, not the physical stuff—she knew more than she wanted to about *that*. But the conversation they'd had. What was the terrible secret that Francesca had been keeping from Krish? Stella was dying to know. A hidden love child? Multiple personalities? A previous marriage to a serial killer? Her imagination ran wild.

'I'd love to be away within the next hour,' Krish said. 'Stella, I know you're keen to get back to Grace and Connor.'

That, she was. She still hadn't received many texts from her husband; however, Claudia had confirmed that Grace only came to her house on the Friday. A good sign, at least.

'Ah, coffee,' said Krish. 'I'm going to need some of that.'

STELLA DRAGGED HER CAMERA BAG UP THE FRONT STEPS OF HER HOUSE. Two days of carrying it around had made her muscles ache. While having a baby and travelling the world, she'd lost the stamina she'd had working as a wedding photographer. Reaching the top, she unlocked the door, pushed it open, and called out, 'Hell-oooo! Anybody home?'

No reply, but she could hear the distant sound of a big piggy saying, 'I'm a bit of an expert.' She smiled and slid her keys onto a coat hook, dropping her bags near the stairs. A brief glance showed her that Connor still had not put up the gates as she'd asked him to. Her smile faltered.

She turned into the TV room, expecting to see Connor and Grace snuggled up on the sofa watching Peppa Pig together, but they weren't there. Retracing her steps to the hallway, she walked through the dining room and into the kitchen, where she found Connor sitting at the island, laptop open in front of him and headphones on. The shadow of a beard emphasised his jawline, which had the effect of making him even more ruggedly handsome. Grace was sitting on the floor with an iPad. Stella stuck her tongue into her cheek. This wasn't exactly the father-daughter time she had envisaged.

'Connor? Hello?' she said, tilting sideways into his line off vision.

He noticed her and shook his head as though waking up. 'Yay! Mummy's home!' He removed his headphones and scooped up Grace, who screamed *Piggy!* and started to cry. 'Say hi to mummy!' With his free arm, he hugged Stella and kissed her on the cheek, simultaneously passing Grace to her. It was a deft move. 'We missed you. How'd it go?'

Screaming in Stella's ear, Grace straightened her body, making it difficult for Stella to hold on to her. Stella could feel her own blood pressure rising. As far as homecomings went, this was pretty shit.

Giving up on trying to hold Grace, she let her daughter slide to the floor and crawl back to the iPad.

Stella knew where that iPad would be going tomorrow.

'It was fine. Just like riding a bike,' she said a little flatly, wondering if he'd notice her tone. She didn't want to have a fight in front of Grace, but she also wanted him to pick up that something was off.

He continued to type.

She snatched an orange out of the fruit bowl and dug a nail into the rigid flesh, tearing at the rind. 'I'd forgotten how tiring weddings are, but I took some amazing shots.' She'd scrolled through all the memory cards on the drive home, just to check that her images were as good as she thought they were. They were absolutely *bangin'*, to use a Welsh phrase—especially her photos of the bride, which confirmed her thoughts about where she wanted to go with her career. Her time with Ishani had been her favourite. While the wedding exhausted her, it also energised her creatively. It had everything a photographer could want: the luxury location, the gorgeous couple, and the high-spec production design.

'Glad to hear it,' said Connor. He seemed to be reading something on his screen.

'All good here?' Stella slid a quarter of the orange in her mouth and looked around to see if there happened to be an open bottle of wine anywhere. She suddenly needed a drink.

'Um, yeah. Grace has been a dream. Haven't you, Gracie?' he said to the floor.

*Snort*, went the little piggy.

'What did you get up to?' Stella eyed the pile of dirty dishes in the sink, next to a take-away box. So much for the healthy frozen dinners she'd prepared.

'Nothing much. Just hung around here mostly.'

'And Claudia's,' she said sharply.

He didn't notice. 'Oh yeah, she really helped me out. Good ol' Clauds.'

She chewed on another piece of orange, tired of ignoring the elephant in the room. 'What was the big work emergency anyway?'

'The interviews. You know that,' he said with a hint of pique in his voice. At least it meant he was paying attention.

'I thought you'd cancelled your interviews. To spend time with Grace,' Stella said, spitting a couple of seeds into her palm and chucking them in the compost bin.

'I cancelled the less promising ones and moved the others into one afternoon. I need to find a new assistant ASAP.'

She hated how he made it sound like she was being unreasonable. Heat prickled her chest, but then she remembered Grace's presence on the floor and took a deep breath. 'So did you find one, then?'

'Um...yes.' He squinted at something on his screen. 'Actually, no.

Sorry, got distracted. No, not yet. But I'm considering one of the candidates. I still want to see a few more before making a decision.'

'I guess Krish is a hard act to follow.'

'You're not joking.'

A wave of tiredness washed over her, and she decided to pursue this another time. She didn't have the energy for this. Instead, she bent forward and leaned her elbows on the countertop. 'Which reminds me. Do I have a story for you!'

This time, he was busy reading something on his phone. Surely he'd want to know about Krish's non-proposal and break-up with Jess. 'Connor?' she repeated, 'I said I have—'

'YES!' He punched the air and leapt off the stool.

She perked up, his exuberance infectious. 'Good news?'

His mouth turned up into the sexy half smile that she'd loved since day one. 'I've got a meeting with a *Vogue* picture editor on Thursday.'

Clapping her hands together, she said, 'Amazing! That was quick. I didn't even know you were at that stage. How did it happen?'

'Just…connections.' He picked up his phone. 'It's all who you know. That's what my dad always said, and for once, he was right.'

Armstrong also said that marriage was for the weak, so she wasn't too keen on Connor quoting him. 'Shall I open some champagne?' Stella asked as she took two flutes down from the cupboard.

'Can't. Sorry. I have so much prep work to do for the meeting. I've got to put together mood boards, clear my schedule. Oh, I should mention that, if I get this job, I'll need to head to South Africa for two weeks.'

She put the flutes back in the cupboard with a little more force than necessary. 'What? When?'

'End of the month. Hey, maybe it would be a good time for you to go see your parents?'

Convenient. Connor loved any excuse to get out of visiting Wales, even though her mother adored him and treated him like a prince whenever they went. 'Maybe we could come with you. To

South Africa.' She'd love to go travelling with him again. They'd only been back a month, but she could use another dose of the constant adventure.

'Mmm. I don't think so. It won't be any fun for you. I'm going to be working the whole time.'

'That's okay. Grace and I could just hang out at the hotel. Or if it's near Cape Town, we can go to the beach...'

'I just don't think it's a good idea. I'll need to concentrate on the job. It's my first break into fashion, and it's got to go perfectly. Sorry, Price.'

'Oh. Oh, well.' The air in the kitchen became thick with disappointment—not that he noticed—and Stella needed to get outside. 'Come on, Gracie. Let's go for a walk.' It was time for Grace's afternoon snooze anyway. She walked around the island and bent to take the iPad. As soon as it disappeared, Grace started crying.

'Connor, can you help?' Stella pointed her chin towards the pram parked in the corner.

'Of course.' He leapt up to retrieve the pram. Between them, they managed to secure a resistant Grace in the baby seat.

Remembering that she hadn't told him the big story from the wedding, Stella said, 'By the way, Krish and Jess broke up.'

That seemed to get his attention. 'What?! I thought he proposed to her. Paris...wasn't it?'

Stella tucked a blanket into the pram, and Grace tossed it on the floor, still missing her pig programme. 'I guess not. He realised that he didn't want to spend his life with her.'

'Huh. I thought they were solid. I guess you never can tell what goes on behind closed doors.'

As Stella manoeuvred the pram down the front steps, she thought she couldn't agree more.

## 30

FRANCESCA STARTED REMOVING her clothes before they'd even stepped across the threshold of Krish's flat. Now that they'd started having sex, she wanted to get her fill. After all, she could only really engage in intercourse during the first couple weeks of her body's strict schedule of pain and torture, so she wanted to get it in while she could. No pun intended.

They didn't make it past the blue sofa the first time. Second was in the shower. Third in the bed, after which they promptly fell asleep. They didn't awaken until early on Monday, when Francesca slid beneath the covers and woke him up in the best way possible. She could get used to this morning routine.

'Fancy a cuppa?' she said afterwards.

'I'll get it.'

'No, you stay in bed.' She pretended to bow as she backed out of the room naked. 'I can boil a kettle.'

The new-build kitchen was compact but sleek, with a wall of white cupboards and drawers that gave her no hints as to their contents. She opened one and found plates. Another contained wine glasses. Finally she found the mugs—all white as well. She filled the kettle and leaned on the marble counter to survey Krish's man cave while waiting for the water to boil.

It looked like the sort of flat he'd have. Uncluttered, tastefully decorated, just enough furniture. On the wall opposite hung three vintage movie posters: *King Kong*, *Johny Mera Naam*, and the *Blade Runner* one that used to hang above his bed. She smiled. She looked forward to five years' worth of catching up on their favourite films.

The kettle whistled and she poured water into their mugs, making sure to keep the strings of the tea bag from slipping into the boiling liquid. She opened a drawer, searching for a spoon.

A framed picture of Jess and Krish stared back at her. Her smile slipped.

He'd obviously put his couple photos away after the break up. Francesca pursed her lips. The two of them made such a striking pair. What if *they* were meant to be together? Had Francesca fucked up Krish's destiny? What if he decided he didn't want Francesca and her baggage? He could probably still patch things up with Jess, as Ankita had said.

*Stop it*, she scolded herself. *He wants you*.

However, the picture in the drawer reminded her he'd only just broken up with Jess. Glancing towards the bedroom door, she worried that she'd jumped too quickly into Couple Land with Krish. What if she was the rebound relationship? He hadn't really had a chance to consider what being with Francesca meant for his life. He needed to spend some time playing it out, understanding the full consequences. She didn't want to invest in this relationship, only to find that two years down the road, he changed his mind.

'Need any help?' Krish called out.

'Um, no! All good.' She closed that drawer and opened the next one, where she found the spoons.

After splashing milk into his tea and giving it a stir, she added some cold water to cool them down and carried the mugs back to the bedroom, absently humming the catchy theme from one of her favourite Hindi films.

She handed him the mug and crawled back under the covers. He put his tea on top of a book on his bedside table and rolled towards her, propping himself up on one hand, while she settled upright against some pillows.

'So I take it you're a *bahut bada* Bollywood fan now,' he said in an exaggerated accent.

'Well, Bollywood is jolly good.' She blew into her mug.

He laughed at her reference. 'I never, ever would have believed it possible. Not in a thousand years. So what's your favourite?'

'*Mohabbaten*. I'm a sucker for a Shah Rukh Khan film. He really has improved with age. Frankly, I think he's better looking now than he was in *DDLJ*.'

He flicked her on the leg with feigned jealousy. 'He's old enough to be your father. I love the *Dhoom* movies.'

'Criminals with fast motorbikes? *Quelle surprise.*'

'And did you know there's a movie named after me?' He reached out and walked his fingers along her hip.

'Of course! You're a sexy superhero…'

'…with an incredibly high IQ, unbelievable strength, and excellent stamina.' He waggled his eyebrows suggestively.

'Oh, I agree. *Superhuman* stamina.'

He leaned over to trail kisses down her arm. 'I know a good way to test it…'

She laughed, and hot tea splashed over the side of her cup onto her belly, a few inches above one of her scars. 'Shit.'

'Sorry! Did it burn you?' He soaked the tea up with the bed sheet and kissed the spot. Pulling back, he trailed his finger over the puckered skin below. 'When did you get this one?'

'Three years ago. Myomectomy.'

'What's that?'

'Fibroid surgery. Didn't help. They came back.'

Both of them were quiet as he continued to stroke her scar, like he wished he could take it away. Sweet Krish. She wished he did have super powers. If anyone deserved them, it was him. He'd be such a force for good. She knew that he would do everything he could to protect her.

Or to heal her. But of course, that was impossible. Her body was what it was. She'd had over a decade to get used to her problems and what they meant. For him, the entire thing was fresh. He might say that he was fine with her having a hysterectomy, but she'd seen the momentary look of shock on his face when she'd told him. She could only imagine what went through his head in that second. What had been going through his head since.

Francesca sipped her tea and said what needed to be said. 'We haven't talked about the fact that I can't have kids.' The next words were harder to say. 'How do you, um, feel about that?'

He rolled over and faced the ceiling, stuffing his hand behind his head. 'I'm still trying to understand what it means.'

She put her mug down on the bedside table and sat up straighter, looking down at him. 'It means what I just said. I can never carry a baby that's half you and half me. That's what it means.'

Another brief flicker of something crossed his face. 'I know that.'

'But have you accepted that?' She held her breath as she awaited his answer.

He sat up, too, piling his pillows behind him and leaning back against the cushioned grey headboard. 'Are you sure there's nothing that we can do? Can we harvest some of your eggs before the operation? Use a surrogate…'

Her head was shaking before he even finished. 'We already tried. I became overstimulated both times.'

'What does that mean?'

'It means it didn't work.' An edge of frustration sharpened her voice. She crossed her arms.

Krish reached over and slowly uncrossed them, taking her hand in his.

'Maybe you just need to try a different clinic…'

Unexpected tears formed behind her eyes, and she commanded

them to go away. She'd cried enough. Still, she snatched her hand away. 'I was afraid of this.'

'No, sorry.' He reached after her, recapturing her hand. 'I didn't mean to say the wrong thing.'

She turned her head towards the opposite wall. 'But you can't help it. You don't know what you don't know.' Swinging her head back to him, she said, with a note of accusation, 'I bet you've already started researching this on your phone every time I leave the room.' He'd probably have a full dossier completed by next weekend.

'No...' A guilty look turned his lips downwards.

She reached past him and grabbed his phone off the bedside table.

'Okay, YES!' He took the phone back. 'But I just want to learn more about it. We're a team now.'

'Are we?' Her eyes stabbed into his with a direct, no-nonsense intensity.

'Yes! I—' Krish stopped talking, and looked away as though gathering his thoughts before continuing, 'I've already found so much useful information. And read lots of stories about women with these issues who have gone on to get pregnant...'

'I'm getting a hysterectomy in two months.' Her voice struggled to remain calm.

'I know but—'

'I'm just saying it again, in case you didn't believe me the first time.' At the distressed look on his face, she softened and continued in a less agitated voice, 'Listen, this is all new to you, so I'm going to give you some leeway. But don't forget that I've been living with this for years. If I went on Mastermind, female reproductive disorders would be my chosen subject.' She paused for a moment, pondering how she could make him understand. 'How many different specialists do you think I've been to?'

His eyes flicked up, counting imaginary specialists. 'I don't know...ten?'

'Wrong. Over thirty. Gynaecologists, psychologists, pain specialists, gastroenterologists, urologists, dieticians, personal trainers, reflexologists, I could go on...thankfully, my parents pay for private medical, because this all adds up quickly. Managing my symptoms sometimes feels like a full-time job.'

'I read that acupuncture can help...'

She grunted. 'Tried that. Thank you for playing.'

'What about—'

'How many steps is it from your office desk to the toilet?'

He shook his head, surprised by the question. 'I don't know. Fifteen?'

'Eh!' She held her arms up in the shape of an X. 'The answer is forty-two. I know this because I've counted them. I also know that it's five steps in my flat—the benefits of living in a small studio—and ten here. Sometimes that journey feels like a lifetime when my pain is at its worst. Every step is agony.'

'Have you tried medication? Surely there must be something...'

She shook her head, appreciating that he was engaged but also wishing he would stop. 'Krish, I've tried it all! Birth control pills made my boobs hurt, and I put on so much weight. Ditto the coil. Metformin made me feel bloated and gave me stomach cramps. And sugar! The reason I can't eat any cake is because of the headaches. Thank you, PCOS.'

'It's just hard to believe that there aren't more options for you.'

Throwing up her hands, she said, 'Welcome to the great injustice of being a woman. There's so little research into these conditions. That's what happens when men are controlling the budgets and women are discouraged from going into science.' Her voice dripped with anger. This was a well-used, infuriating soap box for her.

He reached for her hand, but she resisted. She had to do what was right for once. 'No, Krish. I think you need to think about this some more. Decide if you really want to be with me and all the baggage that brings. What it means for *your* future.'

'Francesca, I want *you*.' His eyes were so earnest. She wished she could believe he'd really thought this through.

'I want you, too. But I...I care for you too much to subject you to this.' She indicated herself. 'That's why I broke up with you five years ago. You deserve to be a dad. You were practically built for it.'

He stayed silent, neither agreeing nor disagreeing.

The next words killed her, but she said them anyway. 'I think we should take a break.'

Krish snorted. 'Okay, Rachel...'

'No, seriously.'

'But we only just found our way back to each other. Don't do this to me, again, Chezzy.' He drove his hands into his thick hair, his voice thick with anguish.

She hated doing this to him. But it was for the best. Due diligence before embarking on a life shackled to her and her problems. 'Just one week. That's all I'm suggesting. Take a week to really think about it without all of this distracting you.' She swept her hand across the messy sheets. 'Next Sunday, we can get together and talk about what you've decided.'

Eyes narrowed, lips thin, he said, 'One week?'

'Just one week.'

He sighed. She could hear frustration in that sigh. 'Okay. One week.'

Reaching out, she touched his arm. 'Promise me you won't try to contact me?'

An exasperated noise preceded his saying, 'I promise.'

Francesca slapped her hands onto her thighs, probably a little too hard. Better that than tears. 'Right then. I guess that's that. I'll get a taxi home.'

'I can drive you.'

'No, it's okay. I can get home by myself.' She didn't want to draw out this separation any more than it had to be.

He stopped in the process of getting out of the bed and sat back down, turning towards her. 'You know, I think you have some thinking to do, too.'

'I already know what I want.'

'Yes, but if I choose you, will you be able to fully commit to me? Will you listen when I say I want to help you? Most importantly, will you tell me the truth? Always? You can't keep things from me anymore. I need to be able to trust you. No more Normans.'

Her cheeks broke out in a guilty blush, and her chest tightened. 'Do you...do you think you'll ever be able to trust me again?' She had to know.

Krish looked her straight in the eyes. 'I want to.'

That wasn't a yes.

She had already caused him so much pain. She wasn't worthy of this naked superhero who made her world explode with stars when he touched her. With supreme effort, she extricated herself from the sheets, found her clothes, and put them back on. She shoved the rest of her things into her backpack.

Slowly, she trudged to the front door and let herself out. He followed, donning a robe on the way. With the threshold of his flat separating them, he kissed her like it might be their last time. 'Chezzy, I—' He stopped and closed his eyes for a second. 'I'll see you in a week.'

She left in a hurry, before she lost her nerve.

## 31

'DID you know that some women report that period pains feel equivalent to the pain of a heart attack?' Krish said to Mick in the lobby of his office building.

'That sucks,' said Mick, whose thumb was saving his place in a well-worn copy of *Bridget Jones's Diary*. 'Actually, I saw somewhere that male doctors used to tell women not to read because their ovaries would become inflamed.'

'Absolutely crazy,' said Krish. No wonder Francesca had been so angry. She had been right to get frustrated with the lack of knowledge and research into her conditions. He'd read that diagnoses could take anywhere from six to ten years because doctors wrote off women complaining of symptoms as just that: complaining. And things were even bleaker for black and brown women, who—it was only recently discovered—had even *more* severe growths of endometriosis than white women. He was enraged for them all.

Four days had passed since Krish last saw Francesca and, in that time, he had become a walking encyclopaedia of women's reproductive health. He'd learned new words like *prostaglandins* and *dysmenorrhea*. His computer browser had millions of open tabs—something his inner neat freak never normally allowed—as he researched

Francesca's issues. A dedicated notebook was already half-filled with his scribblings and stuffed with print-outs.

The more he read, the more he respected the strength she exhibited just by waking up in the morning and getting out of bed. His warrior woman.

Some people might call his research overkill, but he called it romantic. He loved Francesca, and he wanted to educate himself so he could support her. He'd already put his foot in it a few times and didn't want to be insensitive by accident. If everything worked out, then he wanted to be her partner in every way.

Assuming she chose him, too.

At his flat, the words 'I love you' had almost slipped out a number of times, but something stopped him from saying them. It felt like dangerous territory. The last time he'd said those words, Norman had happened.

Krish realised that he had Norman post-traumatic stress. Every time he heard that name, he needed a deep breath. If...*when* they managed to sort things out, they would have to do something to take the power away from the name Norman. Krish couldn't go through life randomly hating innocent Normans.

But...what if she just didn't believe him when he said that he wanted to be with her? That he'd thought it through?

He understood her reluctance, but that didn't make what she had done okay. Five years ago, she hadn't trusted him enough to be honest; what made him think that she would do so now?

Krish didn't want to get hurt again.

Up in his office, he sidled past Francesca's desk and sighed. The place felt empty without her.

The moment he sat down at his computer, his phone rang. He glanced at the name, hoping it would be her, but it was his brother-in-law. He answered straight away. 'Max, hey! Everything all right?'

'It's happening!'

'The baby?'

'She's on her way! Any minute now. Ankita wanted me to tell you to come to the hospital. Or maybe she just wanted me out of the room because I'm a mess. Either way—' He gave Krish the name of a hospital in Chelsea.

'Okay, I'll be there ASAP.' Krish hung up the phone, grabbed his bag, and ran out the door. 'I'm going to be an uncle!' he shouted to Mick as he shot past.


FRANCESCA SAT ON THE FLOOR IN HER FLAT, DOWNLOADING AND cataloguing footage from the wedding. This would be a huge job. Thankfully, she only had to deliver the teaser reel within six weeks; the rest wouldn't be due for many months. At least she'd have something to keep her busy while she recovered from her operation.

Her eyes shifted towards the kitchen cupboards. King Rat hadn't made an appearance all week. Was it weird that she missed him? She hoped that he had found a better source of food and was living his best life. Francesca didn't want to consider the alternative.

Glancing next to her computer, she perused her To Do list, which covered most of a sheet of A4 paper. In an hour, she had a meeting scheduled with the builder at her old office. She couldn't wait to have that one checked off her list for good.

Another item caught her eye: 'Call gangsta bride'.

*Ugh.* She couldn't put it off any longer. She needed to do it. By contract, the teaser real was due tomorrow. The bride deserved to know all her footage was gone.

Francesca imagined how upset she'd be if she received a call like this. Absolutely devastated. At least thanks to the Blenheim job, she now had funds in her account to refund the couple's money. She just hoped that the bride's dad didn't see this as probable cause to dust off his shovel.

She laughed at the ridiculous turn of her thoughts. Imagine having somebody whacked over a wedding video! No, it would never happen. This wasn't a movie. For things to work out with Krish, she needed to stop jumping to the worst conclusions. If only she had done that five years ago, maybe she and Krish would be married by now. Telling him the truth had lifted a great weight off her. Coming clean with the bride would do the same.

Francesca picked up her phone, and the screen came to life. She tapped the contacts app. The first thing that came up was the last person she'd called: Krish. She'd changed his name back to DO NOT CALL to add an extra layer of protection between her and temptation.

With a determined breath, she closed his file and called the bride. Her stomach muscles fizzled with nervous energy, increasing with every ring. After five rings, she relaxed. Maybe it would go to voice mail.

'Hello?' the bride, Jenny, answered in her sweet, girlish voice.

Francesca tried to make her greeting light and breezy. Dial a smile! 'Hi, Jenny, this is Francesca March.' And when she didn't respond: 'I filmed your wedding?'

'Yes, of course! Great to hear from you! We're, like, *so excited* to see our wedding film. I can barely remember the day, you know? It went so fast.'

The excitement in the bride's voice made Francesca's stomach sink. No turning back now. The only way through was forward. 'About that. I have bad news. My office was burgled, and the footage from your wedding was stolen. I tried to have the files retrieved from the cards, but the technician couldn't do it. I'm afraid...I'm afraid I can't do your wedding video for you. I'm so sorry.'

The bride was silent for a few seconds. Francesca prepared herself for tears, so she was taken aback when the bride screeched, 'Are you fucking kidding me?' like Francesca had just confessed that she'd decapitated her favourite pony. All traces of sweetness were gone.

'As I said, it was out of my hands. I was burgled.' Francesca kept her tone calm, logical.

With a tinge of hysteria, the bride said: 'You *do* know that my husband is a lawyer?' *And my father is a notorious murderer*, Francesca

284

filled in. 'We're going to sue the pants off you.' *And murder you in your sleep.*

Determined to keep it professional, Francesca stated, 'I understand you're upset, but if you look at the contract, damages are limited to a full refund, which I'm happy to give—'

The bride barked a cruel laugh, and Francesca shivered, wondering if Jenny had inherited that from her dad, Chuckles. A vision of him chortling like a maniac as he piled dirt on bodies flashed through her head.

Jenny said, 'I'm going to tank your reviews. I'll ask everyone I know to give you one star.'

Francesca didn't rise to it, as she might have in the past. Jenny was just angry and lashing out. If Francesca were in her shoes, she'd probably be in a rage, too. 'All I can say is I'm sorry.'

'Damned right you'll be sorry. Just wait til I tell daddy. He's going to be *furious.*'

The words rolled so easily off Jenny's tongue, turning Francesca's blood to ice. Jenny must have been using her dad as a threat all her life. Somebody pushed her over in the playground? *Wait til I tell daddy.* Boyfriend broke up with her by text? *Wait til I tell daddy.* Videographer lost all her wedding footage?

*Wait til I tell daddy.*

A bead of sweat dripped down Francesca's forehead, and she wiped at it with her sleeve. In a soothing tone, she said, 'Okay, well, let's not do anything—'

'You better watch your back, bitch.' Jenny hung up.

For a moment, Francesca just stared at her phone, her heart thumping erratically and her imagination running wild. She could see the scene now:


FADE IN:
INT. A MASCULINE HOME LIBRARY - DAY.
Hard lines of dusty sunlight enter through slatted blinds. A

Victorian mahogany executive desk dominates the room. A man known as CHUCKLES (65) sits behind the desk in a leather armchair, smoking a cigar. JENNY (25), his daughter, runs into the room, crying. He stands and she falls into his arms.

JENNY

Daddy, my videographer lost all the footage from my wedding. Will you kill her for me?

CHUCKLES

No problem, sugar. She'll rue the day she crossed the Bonneface Family. Anyone seen my shovel?

Perhaps they could use a better scriptwriter, but the gist was there.

Would Jenny's dad really do something to her over a wedding video? Remove a finger? Break an arm or even a leg? Worse…

The nightmare played out in her mind: the soft, repetitive footfall of an assassin, a red laser appearing on her chest, the James-Bondesque chase over the rooftops of London, ending with her body falling to the paving stones below as a crowd gathers and some tourist from New York mutters, 'And they say *our* city's dangerous!'

She squeezed her eyes shut and shook her head vehemently. *No way*. Chuckles wouldn't risk going back to jail over a *wedding video*. The idea was ludicrous.

…Wasn't it?

Krish's face cut across her thoughts. Should she call him? Just to let him know what had happened? Get his advice…?

Francesca's finger navigated to DO NOT CALL and hovered a millimetre over the keypad.

No. She was just using this as an excuse because she craved his voice. She'd promised him space to think, and she couldn't break that promise over this. Besides, even if she were in real danger,

Chuckles didn't know where she lived. She could just hide out here until Sunday, when she could see Krish again.

The alarm on her phone went off, making her jump. She almost forgot that she had to go to the office to meet the builder in fifteen minutes.

How fast could someone order a hit? Surely, it wasn't an on-demand service, like Deliveroo. She'd have time to sneak out to the office, do what she needed to do, and sneak back, long before any assassin had time to do the necessary groundwork and formulate a plan of attack. She'd seen *Leon the Professional*; she knew how it worked.

Francesca laughed at herself. Of course, the old man who'd tried to hug her at the end of the wedding wouldn't kill her. Would he?

Her eyes slashed towards the abandoned cricket bat leaning in the corner. Not a bad idea to bring it along, just in case.

'Say hello to my little friend,' she said in a really bad Cuban accent.


STELLA SAT ON THE FLOOR OF GRACE'S ROOM, FOLDING LAUNDRY. SHE loved the smell of freshly washed clothes, and she still got a tremor of joy when she saw Grace's miniature outfits. Little shirts, little dresses, little socks. It was hard to believe that Grace would one day be too big for them.

Her daughter gurgled where she was gnawing on wooden rings near the door, chin and chest wet with drool. The white bud of another new tooth had popped through her gums that morning, so it was Calpol and chew toy time.

Stella folded another dress. A strappy number printed with pineapples. So cute.

On the dresser, her eye caught on a photo she had framed from their trip: her, Connor, and Grace standing together in front of the blossoming cherry trees in Japan. It reminded her of that time Connor photographed her in the orchard at the French chateau, surrounded by pink flowers. She smiled. That was four and a half years ago. A lot had happened since.

That morning, he'd left for his meeting with the picture editor at 11:30. They were meeting for lunch at the Connaught. She glanced at her watch. Two hours ago, in fact. He had projected his usual confidence, but she knew him better than that. Inside, he'd be nervous. She gave him an extra big kiss and wished him good luck.

Keen to hear any news, she picked up her phone and texted him.

She checked her emails while she had her phone in hand. Was she hallucinating, or was that an email from Doodlebug Daycare with the subject line: 'Your Nursery Space'? Stella clicked on it and read the text. A place had come up for Grace at the end of the month, and did she want to take it?

The Flash couldn't have written a reply faster than her saying yes.

'Whoop! Whoop!' she cried out. 'Grace, you're going to Doodlebug!' Stella looked at the spot where Grace had been chewing the toys a moment ago. She was gone.

'Grace?' Stella pushed the laundry off her lap. Silence answered back.

Suddenly, something thumped rapidly down the stairs. 'Grace!' Stella screamed and ran into the hallway, gripping the bannister in a hard fist, the air crystallising in her lungs.

On the floor below lay the still form of her daughter.

## 32

Sitting on the edge of the hospital bed, Krish cradled the yellow-wrapped bundle of his new niece in his arms. He gazed into her surprised, dark eyes set in her squashed froggy face. The trademark Kapadia black hair already covered her head. Her arms paddled at the air with jerky movements, as though trying to figure out where all that warm amniotic fluid had gone. He caught her tiny fist between his fingers, kissed the flaky skin, and wiggled his pinky into her strong grip.

It had taken him less than a second to fall in love with her.

'I'm your favourite uncle, Krish,' he said in a sing-song voice. 'And I'm going to spoil you rotten.'

The baby's wet lips made a sucking motion in response.

'Okay,' said Ankita, lifting her arms like they weighed a tonne, her normally photo-perfect hair lank and heavy with sweat. 'Time to hand her back. Looks like the wretched creature needs another feed.'

He passed her over, accidentally leaning on Ankita's legs as he moved away. 'Sorry!' he said with concern. She didn't need her 200+ pound brother crushing her.

'It's fine,' Ankita said as she helped the baby latch onto her breast. 'The joys of a c-section. I can't feel anything below the waist.'

'I have never been so happy that I am not a woman,' said Max from a nearby chair, still wearing a hospital gown, his haunted blue eyes focused on a scene no one else could see.

'Women are warriors,' said Krish. 'They put up with so much more than we can even imagine.'

'How long does this *bleeding* go on for?' Max asked, eyeing up the stack of thick feminine hygiene pads next to the bed.

'Six weeks,' said Ankita, and Max blew out a long breath, shaking his blond head.

Krish had a fun fact for just this situation, thanks to his recent research. 'Did you know that women lose anywhere from two table-spoons to half a cup of blood during each period?'

Ankita huffed. 'Is that all? Feels more like a litre.'

Max shivered. Krish knew that, as one of six brothers, Max hadn't grown up with heaps of female influence.

'Darling,' said Ankita. 'Isn't it time for you to get some lunch? Or dinner? Or anything? Just go away, okay.'

She didn't have to tell him twice.

For a moment, both Krish and Ankita stared at the baby's bobbing hairy head as she sucked away, soppy smiles on their faces. Ankita moved her eyes to Krish and said, 'I wanted to say sorry about the other day…at the wedding. It's just…when I saw you with *that woman*—'

'Francesca.'

'*Francesca*,' she said with great effort, 'I saw red. You know how I feel about her.'

He made sure to catch her gaze when he said, 'What's important is how *I* feel about her.'

She paused for a moment, puckering her lips and rolling her tongue around her mouth. The Ankita thinking face. 'Okay, then. How do you feel about her?'

The words came easily to him. 'I love her.'

She made a pffff noise.

'Big, there's stuff you don't know.'

'Tell me then.'

He stopped and considered whether to share what he knew about Francesca. He didn't want his sister to hate her. If he was going to be with Francesca, then he couldn't keep them away from each other. He loved them both. And he especially loved the little nugget in Ankita's arms.

So he told her. He explained that Francesca had fertility issues and that the fact she couldn't have kids made her think that he was better off without her. He also mentioned her family and how they had always made her feel lesser. He had never really understood her relationship with them until now, but as he explained it, everything Francesca had ever said about her family made sudden sense, reframed by his new knowledge.

Poor Francesca. He had the urge to rush over to her flat.

'Let me get this straight,' Ankita said as she switched the baby to her other breast while Krish averted his eyes, 'she *lied* to you, made up a boyfriend, broke your heart, and now you want to pretend like that's all okay?'

'Try putting yourself in her shoes, Big. She was afraid. I know that's a foreign emotion to you, but...try.'

'I don't know. You still need to think about this long and hard. If you end up marrying her, then you'll never have *this*.' She indicated the suckling at her chest.

His voice rose with unintended anger. 'You do know there are other ways to have a family, right? And if we do, we do. And if we don't, then we just don't. I don't *need* a child to qualify my life. My ego isn't so big that I feel I need to fill the world with tiny Krishes.'

Their eyes battled in a mutual stand-off, as they had many other times throughout their lives. However, none of those times felt half as important as this one. He stared harder. Her lips quirked to the side. Finally, she said, 'I beg to differ. The world needs more people like you, Little.'

And he knew that was the closest she'd come to admitting she was wrong (god forbid), at least for now. Besides, he didn't want to fight with her after she'd just given birth to the cutest baby in the world.

The sound of his phone ringing cut through the silence of the private room. For a brief second he hoped it was Francesca. He was aching to see her.

But it was Stella. 'Krish?' He could hear the desperate tears in her voice. 'I can't find Connor.'

'Stella, what's happened?'

'It's Grace. She fell down the stairs. I'm at the hospital with her now.'

He stood up, alert. 'Oh my god! Is she okay?'

'I don't know. They're checking her for concussion. But I've tried calling Connor, and he's nowhere to be found.'

Krish thought for a second. 'Did you ping his phone?'

'Yes, but it's turned off.'

Strange. Connor never turned off his phone.

Stella explained, 'He had a meeting with a picture editor from *Vogue* today, but that should have ended hours ago.'

Those words twigged something in his memory, but he couldn't put his finger on what it was. 'Okay, send me the address of where you are and I'll see if I can track him down.'

'Thank you, Krish. You're a good friend.'

'And Stella, don't worry. Grace will be okay.' He hung up and hoped it was true. To Ankita, he said. 'I have to go.'

'I gathered. Go, go!'

His phone dinged with the address of the hospital. It was on the other side of town near the Knights' home in Little Venice.

Where could Connor be?

Krish called his ex-boss' number and had the same result as Stella. But he still had access to Connor's diary, and he checked the entry for today. It said: Pic Ed Vogue/VV and the location was set to the Connaught Hotel.

Mayfair.

That wasn't too far away. He could get there in half an hour if he jogged to the tube. No point taking a taxi in the London traffic. The streets were engorged with cars. He set off.

RUNNING INTO THE LOBBY OF THE CONNAUGHT, KRISH TURNED towards the restaurant. Ignoring the calls of the hostess, he cast his eyes over the tables, searching for Connor. It was mid-afternoon, so it wasn't too full.

No Connor.

He turned to the hostess so quickly that she took a step back.

'Was there a man here? Good looking, dark hair, grey eyes. Wait, I can show you a picture.' He scrolled through his phone and found a selfie of Connor and him from a wedding last year. 'This is him.'

She considered the photo for a second. Krish could tell the moment she recognised him. Her eyes glazed slightly and she tugged on the end of her long platinum ponytail. 'Oh, yes. I remember him.'

'Is he still here?'

'I can't tell you that.'

He rolled his eyes towards the ceiling and grunted with frustration. She was just doing her job, but he resented it anyway. 'Listen, his daughter has fallen down the stairs, and she's at the hospital. His wife is trying desperately to get in touch with him, but his phone is off. I need to find him. Please.'

She pursed her perfectly-outlined lips and said, 'They left hours ago.'

'They? Who was with him?'

'Um, two women. One in a black suit. Designer. Beautiful afro.'

'And the other?'

'Blonde, tall, great boobs, gold Alexander McQueen dress. Killer heels.'

Realisation hit Krish. Of course. Connor had mentioned the picture editor from *Vogue* after the shoot with Valentina Vavilek. Something about how Valentina was going to recommend him to her friend.

But Stella had told him not to have anything to do with Valentina. Would Connor break his word to his wife? A surprising jolt of anger rushed through him.

'Thank you,' he said to the hostess.

'Good luck,' she said. 'I hope you find him.'

Valentina's house was nearby. It was the only place he could think to check. And the only reason that Krish could come up with for Connor turning off his phone...

...So that Stella couldn't track him there.

Krish took off at a run.

## 33

THE ANTISEPTIC, latex smell of the children's ward filled Stella's nose as she leaned on Claudia's shoulder, watching the doctor examine Grace.

'She'll be okay,' said her best friend. 'My boys fell down the stairs many times. They just bounce at that age.'

That didn't make Stella feel better.

She checked the time on her phone. Four o'clock. Krish had texted forty-five minutes ago to say he'd found Connor and they were on their way. He didn't say where he'd found him.

Urgent footsteps thwacked the linoleum floor behind her.

'Stella!'

At the sound of Connor's voice, she turned and found herself immediately wrapped in his arms. The tears she'd been holding back in front of Claudia came pouring out of her, marking the lapel of his dark blue suit. He held her close, stroking one hand down the back of her head.

'Shhh, shhhh. I'm here now.'

She breathed deeply to calm herself and was immediately struck by the cloying, floral smell of a foreign perfume infused in the fibres of Connor's clothing.

Pulling away, her eyes flew to his face, his attention focused on Grace. Where had he been? How badly did he want this fashion job?

'How is she, doctor?' he said, not registering the change in Stella's expression. She filed it away for later. Their daughter's health was the most important thing right now.

Claudia handed her a tissue, which she took gratefully.

The doctor, who had been quietly getting on with her job while Stella and Connor had their reunion, said, 'I think she'll be fine. I don't believe she's concussed. She has a few bruises and a cut, but other than that—all okay.'

Both parents sagged with relief. 'Thank you, doctor,' said Connor, putting his arm around Stella's shoulders. If he felt her stiffen a little, he didn't let on.

'That being said, I want to keep her in for one more hour, just to observe her, but assuming all is well, we'll discharge her then.' She smiled and left the room.

Stella and Connor rushed to Grace. 'How's my girl?' Connor leaned over to kiss her on the cheek.

'Piggy,' she said, pointing at a Peppa Pig mobile stuck to the ceiling. Everyone tittered with relief.

Settling herself onto Grace's examination bed, Stella assumed a calm, polite expression and cleared her throat. 'So Krish, where did you say you found him?'

'Uh...' She would have had to be blind to miss the momentary look of panic on Krish's face.

Suspicion welled up inside of her. 'Connor?'

He rubbed the back of his neck, the gesture he made when he was trying to come up with a good answer. Letting out a reluctant sigh, he said, 'I was at Valentina's house.'

Stella recoiled like he'd slapped her. 'Valentina *Vavilek*? The same Valentina Vavilek who you promised you wouldn't shoot anymore?'

'Oh, shit,' said Claudia.

Connor pursed his lips. 'Technically, it wasn't a shoot.'

'What the fu—' Stella stopped herself from completing the word.

Her heart beat faster. Good thing they were in a hospital, because she felt on the cusp of a major cardiac event. And there might also be a murder.

'Hey!' interrupted Claudia. 'Why don't Krish and I stay with Grace for a few minutes while you two go and have a chat *not in here*?'

With a glance down at Grace's alert face, Stella said, 'Fine. Gracie, mummy and daddy will be back in just a minute.' She stood and left without waiting to see if Connor followed.

In the empty examination room next door, she spun on him and hissed, 'What's going on?'

He held up his hands. 'It's not what you're thinking. First off, let me say that nothing happened.'

Stella crossed her arms. He was wearing a navy suit with a navy shirt. Convenient. Lipstick marks wouldn't turn up on a fabric that dark.

He spread his hands in front of him like it had all been a great misunderstanding. 'The picture editor was her friend. Valentina set up the meeting.'

'Oh, so she had to come for what? Moral support? Footsies?'

'Please, you know Valentina. She's a bored housewife. She just wanted to feel involved in the creative discussion. Actually she had some good ideas.'

Stella's hands went full Italian. 'I don't care if she came up with the cure to cancer during lunch. You didn't tell me she was involved. In fact, you lied to me point blank.'

Shaking his head, he said, 'I didn't lie...'

'By omission. It's the same thing. *Le bugie hanno le gambe corte*, Connor.'

'What does that mean?'

'Lies have short legs,' she said through gritted teeth.

He rolled his eyes. That one move shot her blood pressure through the roof. 'Look, I'm sorry. It was a bad call—'

'You're telling me. So why were you at her house? I thought you were meeting at a restaurant.'

'Well, the good news is that...I got the job. We went back to Valentina's so we could discuss the assignment and go over the ideas with more space, have some champagne...'

'Ha!' Stella threw her head back with the exclamation. 'Please, Valentina was probably hoping for a *ménage a trois*.' She shook her head and slit her eyes to the open door of the examination room. Outside, a mother bounced a baby on her lap on the orange melamine chairs of the waiting room. She was watching them like it was the Saturday matinee.

If she were Claudia, she would have told the woman to mind her own business, but she was Stella. She shut the door.

'Connor, did you sleep with her?' Her voice dropped low.

'No! Of course not. I can't believe you'd ask me that.'

Stella poked him in the chest, her voice rising. 'You break your promises all the time, Connor! Like the stair gate. You promised you'd put it up while I was at the wedding. I asked you a million times to do it. This wouldn't have happened if you'd kept your promise.'

'So this is my fault?' He put his fists on his waist.

She knew it wasn't fair, but she said, 'Yes! You had three days to do it. But you were too busy...texting with Valentina, I guess.'

A dark look passed over his face. 'And what were you doing when this was all happening? Were you on your phone?'

The fact that he'd got it spot on made her pause.

'I knew it,' he said.

'If you must know, I was texting you to see how your meeting went. But of course you didn't get it because you were too busy turning your phone off and being shady with Valentina et al.'

His jaw clenched and he dipped his head back in frustration. 'I told you, nothing happened.' And then, caging her with his grey eyes: 'Don't forget that, between the two of us, I'm the one who's never had an affair with someone who's married. I'm not starting now.'

Rage saturated her in a flash, her flesh turning red, her eyes popping wide. She couldn't believe he'd gone there.

Running his hands over his face and hanging his head, he said, 'I'm sorry, I didn't mean—'

'No! You're just the one who slept with bridesmaids and mothers of the brides and every Scandinavian model with a pulse before I met you.' Hurt chased the rage through her veins. Connor knew the circumstances of her affair. How the fallout had caused her panic attacks for a year. He also knew how hard it had been for her to put it behind her. Tears thickened behind her eyes.

Connor plowed on. 'It's not my fault that Valentina comes onto me all the time.'

'Her and every other woman!'

'Exactly my point!' He pointed at her, then pointed to the world at large. 'I get it All. The. Time. It's exhausting.'

'I'm crying for you.' She crossed her arms and studied the sharps disposal box.

Taking a deep breath, he leaned back onto the examination table, holding the edge with his hands. 'Did you know that the air stewardess on our flight home gave me her number?'

Cutting her head back towards him, she said, 'No.'

'And the wedding planner at the hotel in Cape Town where I did the shoot? She hit on me.'

'That doesn't surprise me. She had her eyes on you from the start.'

He reached out to take her hand, but she pulled it away, not ready for that yet. He sighed and said, 'Do you know why I've been trying so hard to get another assistant? It's because I don't like to shoot without one. For security.'

'Why? Because you don't trust yourself?'

He groaned with frustration. 'No, Stella, because I don't trust *them*. Before you came along, I had an experience where a client got angry with me when I told her I wasn't interested. She convinced her husband that I'd come onto her, which was...not fun to diffuse. After that, I decided I'd *always* have an assistant on shoots with me.'

'You never told me this.'

'It never came up.' He kicked at a stain on the floor.

Out of nowhere, she thought of Wally, how he was judged for his looks, too. Not in the same way as Connor, but not entirely dissimilarly either. Then again, being good looking came with its perks, too. She wasn't completely buying his sob story.

'It doesn't change the fact that you lied to me. And that since we came back, you've been ignoring me unless you want food or sex.'

He studied her for a moment and reached for her hand again. This time she let him take it. 'I'm sorry. I didn't mean to make you feel that way. I just...didn't want to miss this opportunity.'

Letting him see all the sadness she felt through her eyes, she said, 'Was this opportunity more important than being honest with your wife?' A sob caught her unawares. 'Why didn't you trust me to have your back?'

The silence hung between them.

She continued, 'I'm not an idiot, Connor. I wouldn't have made you skip this meeting because of where it came from. I know just as well as you what it could mean for you. For your career.' She turned her head towards the wall and squeezed his hand. 'But we could have worked together to figure out a way through it that sidelined Valentina.'

He raised her hand to his lips and kissed her just above her rings. 'I can only apologise. And say I won't do it again.'

'Okay, well.' She studied their conjoined hands, frozen in an imitation of the day he slipped that wedding ring on her finger. There was so much more to discuss. He needed to change; it wasn't an option. They couldn't go on like this, with her being the invisible wife and him, the star player. She had plans and dreams of her own.

But at this moment they needed to concentrate on Grace. 'I'm not done talking about this,' she said, 'but right now, I want to hold my baby girl.'

She freed her hand, threw open the door, and strode back to Grace's room. But not before noticing how the woman in the waiting room ogled Connor.

Krish wished he hadn't been able to hear every word of Connor and Stella's argument, but he had. The walls in this hospital weren't that thick.

'So...' said Claudia while stroking Grace's arm, 'how'd the proposal go?'

'It didn't.' He hoped she wouldn't ask more. The last thing he wanted to do was launch into that story.

'Oh, well. Sorry to hear that.'

That was surprisingly sensitive for Claudia.

'Kiss,' Grace called to him. She couldn't say his name properly. He thought it was adorable. Picking up her little hand, he nuzzled the palm and then blew a raspberry on her stomach. She giggled.

Yes, she would be fine.

Stella and Connor on the other hand...

As he listened to their argument, something struck him that seemed profound in that moment: a couple having a biological child didn't guarantee any fairy tale endings. People acted like that was the gold standard of families, but it simply wasn't. Families came in all shapes and sizes. Assuming everything was in working order, any man could make a baby. George Lucas was 69 when he had his last child.

But it took a real man to make a relationship work.

## 34

FRANCESCA LOOKED up at the odious building that housed her old office. She shuddered. How had she put up with this place for so long? It stank of urine and made her feel like she was a character in a film where people would scream at the screen: 'Don't go in that room! He's going to kill you!'

After her call with the bride, that scenario seemed uncomfortably more probable than it had before. Her brain flip-flopped between thinking nothing would happen to believing that she was in mortal danger.

One hand held her cricket bat, which she tapped against the side of her calf. Her other hand stroked the bottle of criminal identifier spray in her pocket. She'd bought it from a Facebook ad months ago, but then stuck it in a drawer and never used it. Pepper spray was illegal, so the next best thing was a non-toxic red foam that stuck to criminals' skin. She'd watched a video of somebody testing it, and he said it took him four days to wash off.

For the millionth time since leaving her flat, she surveyed the landscape for tails, just in case. Nothing seemed out of the ordinary, but then again, what did she know? That guy vaping next to the newsagent across the road could be a mob hitman. That old woman with the Zimmer Frame, a trained killer.

Hefting the cricket bat onto her shoulder with a confidence that was all for show, she swaggered towards the door and pushed it open. Breaking into a run, she climbed the stairs two at a time, assuming that a fast target would be harder to hit.

She crashed through the door to her office and the first thing to hit her was the stench. She covered her mouth with her hand. Take-away boxes filled with gnawed bones littered the desks, and crushed cans lay like little aluminium corpses across the floor. Somebody had been squatting here.

Placing her cricket bat on the table, she pulled a bin liner and a pair of yellow gloves out of her backpack, having come prepared for all possibilities. She quickly did what she could before the builder arrived, filling up two bin bags in minutes. The odour of rotting food lingered.

All she could think as she tidied was that she longed to be in Camden, in the office she shared with Krish.

Krish. She missed him so much it ached. The memory of their recent lovemaking replayed through her mind, and she had to stop for a minute to catch her breath (a bad idea in the present stinky situation). She squeezed her knees together to further the pleasant sensations swirling between her thighs. What was he thinking right now? Was he leaning towards her or away? She wasn't sure how she'd survive if he chose a life without her. Between the threat from the bride and the idea of losing Krish, the latter won as the scarier prospect. Life wouldn't be worth living without him, which sounded melodramatic even to her ears. But it was also true.

A door slammed somewhere in the building, and she jumped.

'Hello?' the builder called from down the hall.

'Get a grip, Francesca,' she muttered to herself. 'In here!' She poked her head out the door.

The meeting with the builder was brief. He agreed to do all the work next Tuesday, and it wouldn't be as expensive as she'd thought. Result. One more thing ticked off her list.

After he left, she threw a few more things into rubbish bags, but didn't want to dawdle. Her logical brain and her imagination were still playing tug of war over her current mortality risk. She'd return next week after the work was completed to give it a good scrubbing.

Next week...she tried not to dwell on it. Next week, she'd either be with Krish or she wouldn't. She had to think positively. It's what King Rat would expect.

Gathering up the necks of the bags in her fists, she stepped towards the door and stopped. Some instinct told her to be still. Her ears picked up the distinctive whooshing sound of the front door swinging open, but no bang as it closed. Somebody must be taking great pains to ensure it didn't slam shut. She froze, heart picking up pace.

The slow, measured clack of a man's dress shoe echoed steadily up the stairs. Heel, toe. Heel, toe. A moment later, another joined in, following close behind the first.

She swallowed hard. Two men. Her skin crawled with electrified ants.

At the top of the stairs, they paused.

Francesca stilled her breathing, scared to make even the faintest noise.

The door to her office was ajar thanks to the missing locks. With painful slowness, she released her hold on the bin bags throttled in her sweaty fist. The brief static noise of the plastic settling crackled loud as a gunshot in the small room.

Seconds later, the two pairs of footsteps resumed, heading her way.

Again, Krish's face swam before her eyes. The decision not to call him earlier, or at least tell him where she was going, struck her as the stupidest thing she'd ever done. He was her *person*. The one human she could count on. She'd never really had a person before.

Someone who didn't live in Spain or have their own family to worry about. Someone who would come running if she needed him.

She needed him now.

They said that when you are about to die, your life flashes in front of your eyes. That's not what Francesca found. It was the future that flashed in front of hers: the one she desperately wanted with Krish, but might never have. If she got out of here alive, she was going to show him just how much she loved him. She'd sing it in the streets. Broadcast it on the radio. Spell it out in a field big enough that they could see it in space. She would prove to him that he could trust her. No more hiding.

Francesca set her mouth in a thin, determined line. She must survive. She must live so she could convince Krish to choose her. She would fight. These goons didn't know who they were messing with. She had red spray paint and she wasn't afraid to use it.

She pulled the petite can out of her pocket and positioned her finger over the trigger. Whoever was coming down that hall, they'd better watch out.

With frustration, she eyed the cricket bat, which lay uselessly on the table a few paces away. She could lunge for it, if necessary. But her first method of defence would have to be the spray.

The footsteps came to a sudden stop in front of her door. She was a few feet behind it. They couldn't see her and she couldn't see them. Through the narrow crack between the door's long edge and the door frame, she glimpsed a flash of grey fabric, like a suit. A white hand at the end of a sleeve.

Her eyes widened. This was real. This was happening.

She fixed an image of Krish in her mind.

Blood pounded in her ears.

The door creaked as someone slowly pushed it open. She startled. 'We know you're in here,' said a gruff voice. Easily a killer's voice.

The element of surprise was on her side. It was now or never.

Screaming as loud as her lungs allowed, she jumped over the

plastic bags and aimed her can in their direction. A steady stream of foam shot from her hand like she was SpiderMan.

'What the—?' said the man in front, a short stocky guy with thinning, faded ginger hair and a beer belly. His hand flailed in front of his face, trying to block her attack. Red foam crisscrossed his rotund head. Within moments, he looked like a beetroot with legs.

The second man yelled, 'Stop! Police!'

*Wait, what?* She lifted her finger, which petrified into the shape of a small hook, ready to strike again. She didn't lower her arm. Her whole body shook as adrenaline coursed through her.

'How do I know you're not here to kill me?' she shouted.

The short one, who was scooping foam off his face and shaking it onto the floor, shouted back: 'We're here to get a statement from you. About some hard drives we found in a raid.'

Hard drives...they must have caught the burglars! And even better, they weren't going to kill her! She lowered her arm, tilted her head back, and raised her eyes in thanks to the ceiling.

And then she started laughing.

Once she started, she couldn't stop. She was so overcome with relief that she had to hold her stomach with both arms. Christ on a rollercoaster, it felt good to be alive. She wanted to run right now and find Krish, throw her arms around him, and never let go.

She caught sight of the police man covered in paint. With his bulbous eyes and red skin, he reminded her of a creature from a sci-fi movie. She laughed even harder, tears rolling down her face. The tall one chortled, too, earning himself a withering look from Shorty.

'What? You do look ridiculous,' the taller one said. He didn't have a mark on him. He must have used his partner as a human shield.

'Sorry,' said Francesca, wiping away tears. 'But you did sneak up on me.'

'Are you in the habit of assaulting police officers? We could charge you with possession of an offensive weapon,' said Shorty, examining the effects of the dye on his sausage-like fingers.

That sobered her up. Getting arrested would not be ideal right now.

'Leave it off, Niles,' said the tall one. 'Are you Francesca March?'

She nodded.

'Do you know one Larry Bonneface?'

Her hand went to her throat, and all remaining joviality disappeared. 'You mean Chuckles?'

'So you do know him.'

'Well, we're not mates, if that's what you're asking. I shot his daughter's wedding.'

The detectives exchanged a significant look. 'We found property belonging to you on a raid at his house a few days ago. We've reviewed the material and found incriminating evidence recorded in the audio. He was bragging about at least five unsolved murders that he claimed to have committed.'

'Holy shit.' She shivered. Krish was right. Chuckles had been dangerous. She remembered how he had tried to hug her at the end of the wedding and she'd stomped on his foot by 'accident'. Gangsters killed people for less. 'Is he...is he in custody?'

'Yes, we've got him.'

Even as relief washed through her, something bothered Francesca. 'But I spoke with his daughter earlier. Does she know about this?' Jenny's anger had seemed authentic. But either way, she could forget about that refund.

'No, Bonneface doesn't want his family to know. They think he's no longer involved in crime,' said Shorty.

The tall one pulled a notebook and pen out of his inside jacket pocket. 'Anyways, we just have a few questions.'

It didn't take long for her to answer them, which she did as succinctly and accurately as possible. She didn't want this to last any longer than necessary. After all, she had a boy to win over. Ten minutes later, they wrapped up, taking her phone number in case they needed her again.

'When can I get my hard drives back?' she asked.

'When our investigation is over.'

She assumed that meant 'never'.

After they left, she grabbed her things and the full bin bags, depositing them in the skip. She couldn't wait to take a shower and wash off the past couple hours. She could feel the residue of fear all over her body.

But first...

The desire to tell Krish all about her crazy day made her pull out her phone. She opened her contacts and scrolled to DO NOT CALL. Smiling, she changed it back to KRISH. And then for his last name, she wrote ICE: *In case of emergency*. He was her person, after all.

But did he trust her to be his? She winced. If she could go back in time and do it all again, she would have been honest with him from the beginning. She would have given him the choice. Instead, she'd wasted five years that she could have shared with him and now he rightly didn't trust her with his heart.

How could she show him that she was 100% on Team Krish and Francesca?

Her finger tickled the air over his number. She vibrated with the need to call him.

However, something held her back. Krish deserved more than a phone call. He deserved something bigger, bolder. Their love deserved fireworks and sky-writing and a race through an airport. She wanted to shout her feelings from the rooftops, not put them at the mercy of the airwaves.

And she wanted to be able to see his face while she did it.

No, she needed a better plan. She shoved the phone into her back pocket. What could she do?

She ambled in the direction of her flat, eyes unseeing as she went through a list of possibilities in her head. Unconsciously, she hummed *'Cecilia'*—the song that Krish had sung to her on his ukulele.

Turning the corner, five Golden Retrievers on leads danced

across her path, almost knocking her over. She stumbled against the brick wall. The dogs' owner, a middle-aged man with shaggy grey hair and a fluffy beard, failed to acknowledge her at all, despite the fact that his dogs had practically attacked her.

It was on the tip of her tongue to say, 'The pavement is for everyone, dickhead' when an idea swirled into her brain.

The dogs had inspired her.

It was perfect—exactly the right way for her to show Krish that she was in it for the long run. Now that she'd thought of it, really it was the only way.

She just needed the buy-in of the only person who could help her to execute it.

She slid her phone back out of her pocket and made a call.

KRISH STOPPED IN FRONT OF THE MEETING PLACE AS APPOINTED BY Francesca's text: a bench facing the Thames in Jubilee Gardens, Southbank. She included a pin to mark its exact location, so he knew it was the right one. When he looked at the map, he thought the spot sort of looked like a uterus and fallopian tubes from above. Did she choose it on purpose? Was it a coded message?

Or did he just have uteruses on the brain? Probably the latter.

To his left, the London Eye towered above him; to the right, a striped red and white merry-go-round waited for the first customers of the day. Her instruction told him to to be there at 9:45AM sharp on Sunday morning, before Southbank became stuffed with tourists. That said, there were still a good number of early risers milling about, mostly parents with glassy eyes and children keen to break free of their prams.

He parked himself on the bench, his eyes darting around for Francesca. Too full of nervous energy to make himself comfortable, he leaned forward and rested his elbows on his knees. His foot tapped on the grey paving stones.

What was she going to say to him? Had she chosen a public place because she didn't want a scene when she told him that she'd changed her mind?

A young man settled himself on the bench next to Krish and nodded when they made brief eye contact. He took out a copy of the *Sunday Times* and started reading it.

Krish checked his phone to see if any further instructions had come through. Not a word. He confirmed the time again. Only a few minutes had passed since he last looked.

His foot tapped faster. The closer it got to ten o'clock, the more people turned up. Some had picnic blankets, which they spread out on the grass. Closer to the river, a vendor was setting up a stall with hot nuts for sale. Their honey-roasted, sweet fragrance filled the air. If Krish had to sniff that much longer, he'd jog over and buy some.

A woman pulled a speaker on a trolley into the the space in front of him. She set the speaker down and attempted to pack up the trolley, but it got stuck. He leapt up to help her, glad to have something of use to do. He jiggled the handle until the problem resolved itself. She smiled and said thank you. He returned to his bench where the man still sat.

Krish crossed his arms. Was the woman going to perform a street show? Good. Something to keep his mind entertained while he waited for Francesca.

At bang on ten o'clock, music blared out of the woman's speaker, that familiar Bhangra beat: the whine of the sarangi, the twang of the tumbi and the pluck of the zither accompanied by a woman's plaintive cry. Music he'd been listening to and loving his whole life. He still remembered the first Bollywood film his dad took him to see: *Sholay*. Probably a little violent for a six-year-old, but the characters and sweeping cinematography had stayed with him.

The notes crashed into a driving drum beat. The woman broke into dance, seductively stalking in Krish's direction with her arms waving in the air. The back of one hand slithered down her forearm, repeated on the other side. She winked at him and turned back the way she came. From somewhere, six more women arrived and joined her with the same choreography.

Ah, it was a flash mob. He'd heard of these, but never seen one before. He scanned the area for Francesca, but he couldn't see her anywhere. Shame. She'd love this, especially now that he knew how much she loved Hindi films.

The music sped up, and suddenly ten more people appeared, men and women alike. They were jumping and swinging their arms around. The joy was infectious. Crowds were starting to gather on the grass around the pavement and two little boys attempted to imitate some of the moves. Laughing, Krish turned to smile at the man next to him, but he seemed engrossed in an article about some gangster's arrest.

One song transitioned into another, and the beat changed. More people joined. The man next to him threw his paper down on the bench and ran to the front row, where he started gyrating. Krish laughed. He hadn't even suspected.

In front of his bench, the pavement was now full of dancers, so many that they spilled into the artery paths leading away from the space. It was like sitting in the middle of a West End show. Loads of the performers kept catching his eye, like they were performing just for him. Again, he hunted for Francesca. She really was missing out.

Something about the dance tugged at the back of his memory, like he'd seen it before. One of the participants at the back seemed familiar, too: a man dressed all in black with a thin face and impeccable moves. Nah, it couldn't be.

The music changed again, female and male voices intertwining. The dancers parted, so that a path appeared in the middle of the pavement. A woman in a gold top and gold lycra bottoms drifted down the centre.

Krish did a cartoon double take and his eyes popped out of his head. It was Francesca!

. . .

SKIPPING THROUGH THE CENTRE OF THE DANCERS, FRANCESCA HALTED in front of Krish, trying hard not to reach out and touch him. The look on his face made her want to break down in giggles. What a sight.

Instead, she turned her back to him, slinking her body up and down like she was doing a lap dance. She dropped her chin over her shoulder and winked at him before bouncing back to the others.

Behind her, she could hear Krish's beautiful laughter.

But she couldn't let herself get distracted! This choreography demanded all of her attention. Since she'd called Jaiveer on Thursday, she'd been practising the moves non-stop—the plus side being that it made the time fly by.

Jaiveer had come through. He was rehearsing dancers anyway for the next YRF production, a London/India crossover, so it wasn't too hard to pull something together. He reused some of the bits from the wedding. The only bugger was that Francesca had to pay the dancers £50 each for their time today.

It was worth it just to see that look on Krish's face. Like it was his birthday *and* he'd won the lottery.

The moves flowed through her and her body responded in a way it never had before. For the first time—maybe ever—she was rejoicing in her own physicality. Her left arm worked with her right arm which worked with her right leg which worked with her left leg. And all of them were connected to her heart, which beat with the dual purpose of life and love.

This was her body. Take it or leave it. Yes, it caused her pain and frustration, but it also allowed her to live, love, learn, jump, run and dance. She was alive.

Tomorrow might be another day, but today...today she loved herself.


KRISH'S SHOULDERS MOVED ALONG TO THE MUSIC. HE STILL COULDN'T believe this was all for him.

He had never seen Francesca like this. Whirling and happy, with her arms up in the air and her feet moving like the ground was too hot to stand on for too long. To him, she could have been the only one dancing. His heart beat merrily in his chest.

He loved her. Life would be a never-ending adventure with her by his side.

A new song replaced the old, and Francesca disappeared into the middle of the group. All he could see of her was a flash of gold here and a flash of gold there.

Next thing, she was lifted high onto one of the male dancer's shoulders. The other dancers carried on counterclockwise around her while her partner turned slowly the opposite way. Krish grinned so hard that his face felt like it might crack down the middle.

He wanted this go on forever and wanted it to end as soon as possible. The grass was now covered in onlookers filming the event, and he wished that he'd thought to record it, too. He would never get tired of watching that film.

But then again, experiencing it in real life was good, too. He didn't need a recording to remember his joy as he watched Francesca dancing her heart out.

He could feel the finale coming. The beat of the music sped up; his heart with it. The dancers in front started doing a hook step that involved a shimmying motion on top and then banging their feet on the ground. Row by row, the dancers started copying this move, Francesca glowing with an inner light among them. He was so impressed with how well she was doing, surrounded by what he would call professionals. She blended in perfectly.

There was nothing amateur about Francesca.

The first few rows crouched down, shaking their show hands in Francesca's direction as the final drum beats thwacked through the air. She stood bang in the middle, where Paramjeet and Ishani had stood in the original dance. As the final notes sounded, the company called something out. He couldn't make out what it was.

As quickly as it had appeared, the mass of dancers melted back into the crowds. The original woman reconstructed her trolley and carted the speaker away, like it never happened.

Except it had.

Francesca had done this for him. He hoped that he understood her message.

The only dancer remaining was her. She took a few hesitant steps toward him, her hair damp with the effort of her performance. She had a question in her eyes. He didn't even need her to ask it. He just nodded.

WHEN KRISH NODDED, IT WAS LIKE CUTTING A TAUT ROPE; FRANCESCA ran at him and leapt up into his arms, just like she used to, like she'd wanted to do since he came back into her life.

She wrapped her legs around his middle and her arms circled his neck. In one smooth move, she pressed her lips against his. Everything else disappeared from her consciousness. The crowds, the smell of roasting nuts, the cry of a kid shouting, 'Mummy, what are they doing?'

The only thing in the world was Krish. And he was hers.

Pulling back from the kiss, she found his brown eyes with her green ones and said, 'I choose you.'

It was better than I love you. Choice implied so much more. She was choosing to be with him. Choosing him as her friend. Choosing him as her lover. Choosing him as the person she came home to every night. Choosing him as the one person she shared her soul with.

'I love you, too,' he said.

She whooped, let her head fall back, and yelled out, 'I'm in love with Krish Kapadia!'

'Wow,' he said with a smile as she slid down his body and onto her feet, 'you're really taking to public performance.'

'Listen, I finally got to be the heroine of my own Bollywood movie. I'm going to milk it.'

He laughed. 'Does that make me the hero?'

Taking his hand in hers, Francesca tugged him towards the merry-go-round. 'No, Krish, it makes you my *super*hero.'

# EPILOGUE

## THREE YEARS LATER

CONNOR ORDERED a couple of lagers and went outside to find a table for two in the pub garden. The brick courtyard wasn't busy for a Friday afternoon, and he found a great spot in dappled shade. *Beautiful light*, he thought out of habit.

He checked his Omega watch, a gift from the company when he did a shoot for them. Krish should arrive soon. While Connor waited, he scrolled through the messages on his phone. Nothing from his wife. Loads from stylists, art directors, and picture editors —all regarding upcoming projects. In the next month alone, he had two fashion stories to shoot, along with one wedding and an ad campaign for an established designer brand. Thank the gods of photography that he now had two full-time assistants and a PA to help him run his business, especially since he no longer had Krish or Stella.

Stella…

The love of his life. The bane of his existence.

Okay, that was a bit harsh, but they did have a talent for pushing each other's buttons.

Two years ago, she'd started her own photography company, focusing on glamour portraits of women. He was proud of what

316

she'd achieved in such a short time. Admired her, even. She was approaching the craft in a new way, marrying everything he'd ever taught her about lighting and posing to create exquisite portraits worthy of hanging in an art gallery. She'd started a blog, too, sharing tips and tricks behind the clever things she did: cheap and cheerful ways to create backgrounds, experimental lighting set-ups, make-up tutorials, among other things. Her blog had reached 10,000 viewers a day and she had more social media followers than he did. She had a good thing going.

But they never saw each other.

With his leap into fashion and her success, they gave new meaning to two ships passing in the night. He didn't know how she balanced it all while still being present for Grace, but she managed to be a great mum as well as a busy business woman.

While he felt he was completely failing as a husband and a father.

Two large paws landed on his leg, breaking him out of his thoughts. He gazed into the luminous eyes of a Golden Retriever. 'Hey, Norman!' He dug his fingers into her shiny yellow fur and scratched her neck. Why Krish and Francesca chose to name a female dog Norman was beyond him. 'Who's a gorgeous girl?'

Man, he'd love a dog, but now was not the right time. Perhaps one day, when he retired. Except—he just remembered—Stella had a fear of dogs leftover from her childhood, so there went that idea.

'Hey, boss,' said Krish. Sometimes he still called Connor by his old nickname. It brought a pang to his chest. He missed working with Krish.

'Glad you got the memo about the uniform.' Connor indicated that they were both wearing white t-shirts, khaki shorts, aviator sunglasses, and sandals.

'Ha, well when you spend almost every day with someone for five years, I guess you pick up a few habits.'

'How's business?' Norman decided Connor's feet were the perfect place for a nap. He reached down and scratched her again.

'Great. We just got back from a wedding expo in India. Picked up some huge wedding bookings. Caught up with a matchmaker who's been sending me business. It's all happening.' Krish sipped from his pint and wiped the foam away with the back of his hand.

Connor thumped the table, making Norman lift her head. 'Give my congrats to Francesca for the BAFTA, by the way. That's impressive. I'm impressed.'

Krish smiled proudly as though he'd won the illustrious prize and not his wife. 'Thanks. She worked hard on that documentary. Hopefully it'll help stimulate more spending for research into women's reproductive health.'

'Does she still work with you at all?' Connor had opinions about the pros and cons of working with your spouse.

'Once in a while, but not much. She's freelancing for an endometriosis charity right now, creating content for social media. Interviewing women. Recording their stories. She's found her happy place.'

'Well, pass on my regards.' He liked Francesca. She had a lot of spunk.

Krish sipped his beer. Connor could practically feel the next question coming.

'So, how's Stella?'

Connor rubbed the back of his neck. 'She took Grace and went to Cardiff for a few days to stay with Liliwen. Her husband died a couple months ago. Prostate cancer.'

'Oh, poor Liliwen. I'll send her some flowers.'

A bee landed on the rim of Connor's glass and he wafted it away. He hesitated a moment before sharing, 'She said we need to talk when she gets back.'

Krish leaned forward. 'Sounds ominous.'

'I don't know, Krish...' The words tumbled out of him. 'We don't laugh together anymore. I used to be able to make her laugh.'

'You're both busy...'

'It's more than that. We just don't communicate like we used to.' He lifted his sunglasses and squeezed the bridge of his nose. He suspected that Stella had never really forgiven him for the Valentina Vavilek fiasco three years ago. Even though it was that meeting that gave him his big break. He wouldn't be where he was today without it.

On top of that, they hadn't slept together in over three months, which was a big change from how they'd been in the beginning, christening every surface they could. On their trip around the world, some of those hotel rooms deserved goddamned plaques to commemorate the earth-shattering sex they'd had there. Thank god Grace had been a good sleeper.

Usually, Connor wasn't a sharer about these sorts of things, but Krish was one of the few people he could talk to. Krish knew him and Stella so well, and Krish was probably his best friend, Connor realised. 'I think I'm to blame...you know how focused I get on work.' Sometimes, he scared himself with how focused he could get.

'She's pretty goal-oriented, too. Both of you are the same...once you set your minds on something...'

Connor turned his head, looking away from Krish. 'It's just that she's been...distant lately.'

He didn't want to to bring up that Stella told him she didn't want to have any more children, especially as he knew that Francesca couldn't have kids and they were talking about adopting. When Connor had broached the subject with Stella six months ago, she said she was happy with just Grace and didn't want to go through childbirth again. It made Connor sad for his daughter. Stella was an only child, but he had Michael, his brother, and wanted a sibling for Grace, too.

He worried that what she meant was she didn't want another child with *him*.

How had they come to this?

Perhaps his dad was right. Perhaps the Knight boys just weren't marriage material.

Krish drummed his fingers on the table to snag Connor's attention. 'You'll figure it out, boss. You always do.'

'I hope so. Because god help me, I love her, Krish.'

'Then you have your answer.'

'I suppose I do.' He sighed. *If I could only figure out where to start.* He had no problem putting on the charm offensive with everyone else, but with his wife, she seemed to find it an offensive charm. Things that used to make her laugh now made her mutter in Italian. He couldn't do anything right anymore.

Krish hit the table with his fist, causing Connor to jump and Norman to sniff for danger. 'Don't forget who you are, man. You are Connor *Fucking* Knight.'

*That's right*, he thought. *I am Connor Fucking Knight!* The most awarded wedding photographer in the world, father to a beautiful daughter, husband to a talented wife.

And he knew exactly what he wanted.

## THE END

# AUTHOR'S NOTE

I want to take a moment to acknowledge all the women who live with chronic pain, no matter the source. Women are always expected to just get on with things, no matter how we're feeling on the inside. It can be exhausting.

Everybody's experiences of living with polycystic ovaries, fibroids and/or endometriosis is different. Your cycle will most likely differ from Francesca's. For the sake of authenticity, I based Francesca's cycle on one friend's cycle who suffers from all these issues. I hope that reading about Francesca's journey has made you feel seen.

There are many charities that offer help for women with these conditions.

**In the UK:**
*Endometriosis*
Endometriosis UK
Website: endometriosis-uk.org
Instagram: @endometriosis.uk

*Polycystic Ovary Syndrome*
Verity (PCOS)
Website: verity-pcos.org.uk
Instagram: @veritypcos

*Fibroids*
British Fibroids Trust
Website: britishfibroidtrust.org.uk

## In the US:
*Endometriosis*
The Endometriosis Foundation of America
Website: endofound.org
Instagram: @endofound

*Polycystic Ovary Syndrome*
The National Polycystic Ovary Syndrome Challenge
Website: pcoschallenge.org
Instagram: @pcoschallenge

*Fibroids*
The Fibroid Foundation
Website: fibroidfoundation.org
Instagram: @FibroidFoundation

## More charities around the world:
Canada: The Endometriosis Network (endometriosisnetwork.com)
Canada: PCOS Together (pcos.together.ualberta.ca)
Canada: Vivre 100 Fibromes (vivre100fibromes.ca)
Australia: Fight Endo (www.endofoundationaus.org)

# ACKNOWLEDGMENTS

This is my favourite part to write because it means that the book is done and there will be a party soon.

First, I have to give a shout out to (probably) my best friend, Sarah Gillman. I've watched you deal with the same issues as Francesca for over 20 years. I wanted to write this story as a celebration of all you've achieved and also to try to give others a sense of the hidden pain of these often debilitating issues. I have endometriosis, too, and it blows my mind that there isn't more research into curing this disease. Here's hoping that with more women being encouraged into science and more awareness of the hidden struggles involved, a cure will be found one day.

Many women spoke with me to share their journeys of dealing with polycystic ovaries, fibroids, and endometriosis. You are all brave warriors. I appreciate your honesty.

I had my first taste of Bollywood in 2014 when I was on a bus with 14 other trekkers, heading for the base of Kilimanjaro to begin our 5-day hike to the summit. The driver put on a movie to entertain us. It was called *Krrish 3* and I loved it. Since then, I've had a fascination with Hindi films and, when it came to naming Connor's assistant with leading man good looks, Krish was the name that seemed to fit him best. I hope that Bollywood fans will enjoy the references and those who've never watched a Bollywood film will give it a go. There are loads on Netflix and Prime. As Francesca said, "Bollywood is jolly good."

As ever, I have been blessed with the most amazing group of women in my writing corner. Thank you to Jayne Rice, Juno Goldstone and Farrah Riaz for your beta reading, and Joanna Lyons, Jessica Popplewell, and Amanda Scotland for your encouragement. The J Team's close reading is, as ever, integral to the fabric of this book. This story started on a Curtis Brown Romance course with Jenny Colgan, so thank you to Jenny for helping me to get this one off the ground. And finally, thank you as well to Nicola May for all the encouragement and marketing advice.

To Abhi Parasrampuria, for supplying me with Hindu words, answering my questions, and reading the story despite the fact that romance really isn't his thing. Sima Auntie would be proud.

Big hugs to Amy Borg, editor extraordinaire, and Bailey McGinn, the cover designer with the mostest. I knew we'd get there in the end.

To Roshni Jogia for answering every single question I had about Indian weddings. I have had to take some liberties with the timings. In reality there probably would have been at least a day between the Mehndi Night/Sangeet and the wedding, but I just couldn't keep poor Francesca and Krish hanging on that long. Thank you as well to the staff at Blenheim Palace who answered all my questions when I came for the tour. I know I've taken a few liberties with allowing my photography team to base itself in the staff room below stairs and, of course, the Oberois would either have been close friends of the Marlboroughs to be allowed use of the private apartments or perhaps they just threw a lot of money at it, like Sylvester Stallone.

Veruschka Baudo, *grazie mille* for the Italian corrections. Nick Mervin, thank you for our chat about Scotland Yard. Unfortunately, Francesca's scene there got cut, but I am grateful for the info anyway. I'll tuck it away for the future.

To my readers, I am so incredibly thankful for you. You reading this book is a dream come true for me. I've peppered two *Dirty Dancing* references into this story (there is one in *Shooters*, too). Did you find them?

Huge appreciation to my photography crew for supporting the launch of *Chasing the Light*. James Musselwhite, you are my favourite brainstorming partner. Sanjay Jogia, thank you for the Indian wedding insights. And my everlasting gratitude to: Damian McGillicuddy, Kelly Brown, Gary Hughes, Claire Louise, Fiona ingvarsson, Angela Adams, Maria Michael, Melody Smith, Selena Rollason, Magdalena Sienicka, Veruschka Baudo, Keith White, David Anthony Williams, Tatiana Lumiere, Christine Selleck Tremoulet, Gary Hill, Kristi Sutton Elias, Tianna Jarrett-Williams, Elli Cassidy, Amanda Chapman-Bruce, Martina Wärenfeldt, Kris Anderson, Steve Scalone, Justine Ungaro, Belinda Richards, Maggie Robinson, Sharron Goodyear, Therese Asplund, Neil Shearer, Gurvir Johal, Carol Oltz, Rachel Thornhill, Christina Lauder, Scott Johnson, Hannah McGregor, and Gerson Lopes.

Thank you to my dad and Faith for being HBM Publishing's US HQ.

And finally, it's not easy living with a writer, so sending all my love to my husband, James, who always shares at least one quality with the leading men I write, and my long-suffering children, G and H. Sorry for all the burned pizzas. Mummy loves you.

## COMING SOON

# Are you worried about Jess?

Stay tuned for Jess in Paris (working title), a Photographers Trilogy novella.

Sign up to my newsletter
in order to be the first to
find out when it's available
AND
get the first three chapters for free.

JuliaBoggio.com/signupctl

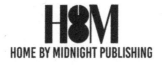

HOME BY MIDNIGHT PUBLISHING

**COMING IN 2024**

# Exposure!

Six months into a trial separation,
Stella and Connor rendezvous
at the world's biggest
photography convention
in Las Vegas.

Can Connor convince Stella
that they can both achieve their dreams
better together than apart?

Not if Blake Romero has his way.

**PRE-ORDER TODAY**

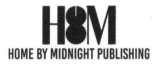

**HOME BY MIDNIGHT PUBLISHING**

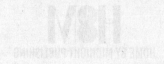

# ABOUT THE AUTHOR

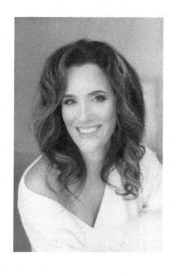

Originally from New Jersey, Julia moved to London in her early twenties. She worked as an advertising copywriter until discovering her love of photography on a 6-month trip around South America. She started a wedding photography business which received some great PR when her own *Dirty Dancing*-themed wedding dance went viral on YouTube. She appeared on *Richard & Judy* and *The Oprah Winfrey Show*, where she danced with Patrick Swayze. In 2009 she opened a luxury portrait studio and has photographed everyone from the Queen to Queen, the band. After 15 years as a photographer, she returned to her first love: writing. Julia lives in Wimbledon with her Welsh husband, two children, and an oddly possessive cat. Sign up for Julia's newsletter at JuliaBoggio.com/signupctl.

Milton Keynes UK
Ingram Content Group UK Ltd.
UKHW042338170823
427067UK00004B/169

9 781739 215132